Cover photo and design: Mario Garrett
Silver Sands, San Diego 2016

IMMORTALITY
WITH A LIFETIME GUARANTEE:
Aging as a Human Survival Strategy

Mario D. Garrett Ph.D.
Professor of Gerontology

Printed in the United States of America

ISBN-13: 978-1545288320
ISBN-10: 1545288321
BISAC: Health & Fitness / Longevity

Published by Createspace, USA

Suggested Citation: Garrett M.D. (2017) Immortality With a Lifetime Guarantee. Createspace. USA.

Acknowledgement

Writing consolidates multiple discussions across a number of years. Discussions with friends, students and colleagues that result in the formation of a number of ideas, some of which made it into this book. This is where I recognize some of these individuals.

Pedram Salimpour inadvertently set me off on this magic carpet of a journey that took me more than eleven years to complete. I am beginning to enjoy the journey more than the destination. My eldest daughter Tabitha Garrett edited versions of this book and provided critical arguments along the way. Dave Baldridge contributed editorial finesse, and intelligent feedback. He continues to polish my written work. My discussions with Ramón (Ray) Valle create a linchpin for many of the arguments found here. Dan MacLeod for encouraging me by reading and commenting throughout this process, nudging me delicately. Richard Prince continues to engage me in discussions and his interest in medical advances has provided me with a sounding board for some of these ideas. Soo-Lai Lam has provided constant support for my work, and remains by my side despite everything else that happens in my life. And last but not least the thousand of students that I teach in California, Turkey, Japan, Malta and Canada for their unbiased questions. Their clarity of vision guides my search for answers. It is truly a privilege to teach so many young people. They are our future and we are fortunate to be in such good hands. The highlights of this book, when you come across them, are their praise, shortfalls remain purely my own.

Mario D. Garrett

Preface

The best way to make money is to create a new religion. You register the religion as a charity, and all profits that you make remain untaxed. You have no commercial product to deliver, no liability, no research required, and no constant updates. You give people hope and salvation from their daily worries.

An early morning breakfast with my friend Pedram Salimpour began with this topic in the spring of 2006. It was an open gambit of what usually turns out to be a protracted but animated discussion of the world's woes. On the patio of the Estancia Hotel overlooking Matlahuayl State Marine Reserve, north of La Jolla in San Diego, we sat, two middle-aged bald men lightheartedly lamenting the state of the world, sharing a breakfast, and catching up on a year's worth of news. After some back and forth, we decided that the best type of religion to promote is immortality. With the Baby Boomers maturing, all seeking youth and longevity, this would be an easy sell.

Pharmaceutical companies would join as "Methuselah" patrons. We could sell stuff to people to make them immortal. The public could perhaps join as "Calment" members, these being in-house jokes at the expense of our "clients." We could also give them "a lifetime guarantee," we quipped. We joined in conspiratorial laughter until we realized that it is so preposterous it might work.

It might work. One thing for sure was that there would be no refunds. And that is how I started developing an interest in immortality. I wanted to expose how this fail-safe method for making money ignored science in favor of sound bites. It took me ten years to incrementally develop this witticism into an academic interest and now into this book. Writing remains an organic process and the journey taught me further about the beauty of our biology and the significance of our psychology.

A lot of good books deal with the topic of immortality, although most are selling a new diet, or pills, natural herbal therapy or other commercial products. Some more serious books deal with the mechanics or the demography of aging, including an excellent book on strategies of how not to think about death. But despite these good publications, we desperately needed a measured scientific and comprehensive perspective that explains the complexity of aging research. The story I am about to tell you is a coherent and comprehensive review of the research on aging. The eventual conclusion will hopefully further our discussion that aging comprises an integral part of our survival as a species. That is take-home conclusion.

This story starts with an exploration of our strategy, as humans, to survive. Nature allows immortality so the question is why not us—why not make humans immortal? To answer this question we have to go on a journey that takes us across ecological biology, genetics, neurology and anthropology. This journey allows us to realize that aging is a result of having a large brain. Both aging and a large brain are necessary to nurture our children. From a natural selection perspective, our children are the next in line for the world's test of survival. Our human strategy for survival involves nurturing a few offspring and providing enough care for them to survive. In order to provide enough learning for our children to survive we needed both a large brain, to contain all this information, and a longer life to be able to impart this information. But there is a problem with this strategy.

Our brain also self-reflects, and we become aware of our own impending death. An Adam and Eve story develops that takes us into sociology, psychology, philosophy, genetics and religion. Knowing that we will die conflicts with our belief in a just and orderly world. We eventually have to develop a way to delude ourselves that aging is the culprit and not the answer to our survival as a species. And our story takes a new twist on how immortality first becomes our religion and then becomes a central feature of our psychology. Through anthropology and history we explore mechanisms for denying death.

In reality there are only a few people who live a long time, centenarians—those that are living beyond 100 years of age. Centenarians have an answer for us, that at the end of our life, our body/mind conspires to keep us alive long enough as needed. How long we are needed is up to us.

To our advantage and disadvantage, we are an integral part of our environment. We are not simply a body. We are a constellation of different organisms, alien DNA, bacteria, viruses, and our own DNA that record its own history and modifies itself. All this activity lives in a state of balance in our body. Dancing to a symphony we remain oblivious to. This book explores the symphony. Enjoy the journey.

Mario Garrett
Vancouver, Canada

CHAPTER 6

CHAPTER 7

CHAPTER 8

INDEX

Chapter 1

Immortality All Around Us

The only thing wrong with immortality is that it tends to go on forever, but what's wrong with that, really?

— Herb Caen (1992). *Herb Caen's San Francisco, 1976-1991* Chronicle Books.

Immortality is everywhere. It is so common that we do not see it all around us. The idea of immortality even pervades all of our religions. Immortality surrounds us in nature and yet we are unaware of it, occupies our thoughts, and yet we are oblivious to it. Although impossible to ever measure—it is infinite and never ending—we seem to have an intuitive grasp of its meaning. We do not need to go far to see examples of immortality because examples reside inside us. Take our genes for example.

Genes have made it from that very first human—a true Eve—and will make it to the last human. This is as good as immortality gets. Such impressive longevity has titillated researchers to view genes as the modern version of a soul. This is not as far-fetched as it seems. In 2001, Alex Mauron, a molecular biologist at the University of Geneva, argued that the early scientists looking at genes saw similarities with the Aristotelian concept of *eidos*, which Thomas Aquinas regarded as the "soul." But how can our immutable genes be judged good or bad? It is but luck—or misfortune—of the draw, something that the Hindis know very well. But perhaps our survival serves as our passport for immortality. In the early 1700s, the controversial Irish writer Henry Dodwell held that all souls are material, with a physical substance to the soul, and only a few souls are granted immortality "… by the Pleasure of God to Punish or Reward by its union with the Divine Baptismal Spirit." We can't talk about immortality without bringing religion into the mix. And there lies the rub.

Why immortality is inextricably entwined with religion will prove to be a very good guide for us in our journey. We will revisit religion throughout the story of immortality. At first it seems like a nuisance—science having to deal with religion—until we realize that religion is dependent on the construct of immortality. And like the air that we breathe, sometimes we forget it is there. Immortality is ubiquitous. Take bacteria, which is the most common organism on the planet—after the virus *Pelagibacter ubique,* which lives in the sea. Bacteria has the cleverest DNA—the genetic codes—because instead of having a line of DNA to copy, which results in the tip of the line always missing out from being copied, the DNA of bacteria is circular. Every time it reproduces itself it does not miss copying the end of the DNA as with humans; and therefore the sister cell it produces is a perfect copy. Being masters at replication, bacteria–with the right conditions–can multiply for eternity. But they have nothing on cancer cells.

Cancer cells—we all have them to a certain degree—are errant cells that have learned how to splice genes. Cancer cells have learned the problem with our DNA—that we miss copying the ends of the DNA. This means that after a number of replications the DNA frays and cannot be copied. Cancer cells learned this mistake and they fixed it. Cancer cells exist throughout our body. Most of the time our body identifies and discards them. Other times we are not so lucky. Cancer cells are so proficient at immortality that one line of cancer cells, from a 31-year old Black woman with cervical cancer, Henrietta Lacks, has provided the basis for most pharmacological testing on human cells. The 1951 HeLa lines of cells—taking the first two letters of her name, a form of anonymity—has become so pervasive that in 1967 Stanley Gartler, and later in 1974, Walter Nelson-Rees found that uncontrolled growth of HeLa has dominated as much as one in five laboratory cell lines. Some scientists have described HeLa as its own species—*Helacyton Gartleri*—and a highly successful one at that. Immortality has its drawback: it does not know how to stop. Immortality exists throughout our bodies. It seems that nature knows about immortality and there is no technical reason why humans are mortal. But so far, we have only looked at simple organisms.

Immortality in nature

Immortality in terms of our genes, cancer and bacteria tells us that biology does not need a lifespan—an end point to life. Mortality is not a mistake, since immortality is all around us. And there are immortal beings with us today—alas not humans. The discovery in 1996 by Christian Sommer, a German marine-biology student, of the Benjamin Button jellyfish is one such anomaly. Benjamin Button—referring to the 1922 short story of the same name by F. Scott Fitzgerald, which was made into a 2008 film where the protagonist is born old and slowly becomes increasingly younger as he ages—is the common name given to this jellyfish. In reality the Benjamin Button is a small 4.5-millimeters jellyfish, the size of a chickpea, with the technical name *Turritopsis nutricula*. Although initially discovered in Rapallo, a small city on the Italian Riviera, its best observation is in Shirahama, a touristy white sandy beach town in Wakayama Prefecture, Japan. The beach was created over a 15-year period with 745,000 cubic meters of sand imported from Perth, Australia, 4,700 miles away. As the silence of the resort is broken every few hours by loudspeakers reminding beach goers to leave the beach clean, Shin Kubota is busy breeding these little jellyfish in a 1920s aquarium in Shirahama that is part of the Seto Marine Biological Laboratory, Kyoto University.

This small jellyfish is unique in that it can reverse its life-cycle. Typically, jellyfish die after reproducing, but the *Turritopsis nutricula* enters into a biological loop that cycles from a juvenile polyp to an adult medusa and back to a polyp. Like a Hollywood actor, they go into a cycle from adulthood to childhood. In a personal discussion with Shin Kubota, we do not know whether memory is retained or whether the jellyfish liquidizes itself into a new being. Recent studies suggest that a nerve ring exists that might stay intact throughout this cycle, although Kubota believes that the tentacles hold the secret to its trick of rejuvenation. With the right conditions this jellyfish will keep rejuvenating itself, repeating the loop of life forever.

The strange part of this cycle is that the rejuvenation is brought about by a trauma—in the laboratory produced by fifty jabs with a fine metal pick—from which it responds by amassing its mangled body at the bottom of the sea and rejuvenating itself back to any adult stage. Although immortal, this Benjamin Button jellyfish is still vulnerable to predators such as sea slugs, and they are prone to being suffocated by organic matter, and they can die from lack of food, deformity in its polyp stage and water colder than 72 degrees. As impressive as this jellyfish is, a much more impressive creature exists within this immortality league. Suffering from no such frivolous vulnerabilities, the water bear is not only immortal; it is also ostensibly invulnerable.

The resilient water bear can withstand everything that kills the *Turritopsis nutricula*. The technical name for the water bear is *Tardigrades* (in Italian Tardi Grada meaning "slow stepper"). These little 1-millimeter animals were discovered in 1773 by the German pastor Johann Goeze. *Tardigardes* are animals developed from an embryo stage to an adult with four pairs of legs ending in claws or sucking disks. *Tardigrades* are likely related to insects, spiders, crustaceans, and worms. Including more than 960 species, this small water bear lives across marine, freshwater, and terrestrial environments throughout the world. NASA even sent this creature into space and not only did it survive but during the flight mission, it molted, and females laid eggs. Several of the eggs hatched giving birth to normal newborns. *Tardigrades* can reproduce sexually or asexually. But their passport to immortality is their ability to withstand great trauma. Although *tardigrades* are active only when surrounded by a film of water, they can enter a stage of hibernation in response to: temperatures as low as minus 200 °C (-328 °F) and as high as 151 °C (304 °F); salinity; lack of oxygen; lack of water; levels of X-ray radiation 1000 times the lethal human dose; some noxious chemicals; boiling alcohol; low pressure in a vacuum; and high pressure (up to 6 times the pressure found at the deepest part of the ocean). *Tardigrades* seem invulnerable.

These small creatures, like the Hollywood creation of *The Highlander*, are the archetype of what we mean by immortal: living forever and impervious to trauma. But *tardigrades* offer a more significant lesson for us. Both the jellyfish and the water bear show that biology does not need a lifespan. In exceptional circumstances, biology can create a resilient creature that lives forever without any degradation whatsoever. Aging does not have to result in a weakened biology. We also learn this lesson from animals that live a long time. Although not immortal, such animals have shown how chronological age, passage of time, is not by itself a factor in reduced capacity. These animals show negligible aging.

Negligible Senescence

The concept of negligible senescence—insignificant cell death due to aging—a term used by Caleb Finch with the Davis School of Gerontology at University of Southern California in 1990–describes the extremely slow process of aging in some animals. Using examples from turtles, rockfish, and mammals (especially the naked mole-rat), Finch and others have shown that in some species old age seems to have very little effect on the reproductive success. These animals also evade death for a long time, such as the rougheye rockfish (who can live up to 205 years), sturgeon (150 years for females), giant tortoise (152 years), bivalves and possibly lobsters. Although there is still a lifespan—a prescribed limit to life—negligible senescence shows that reproductive success is not diminished by age alone. Nature has repeatedly shown its capacity to dispel our ideas of aging. It is not necessary for frailty and diminished capacity to accompany age.

Negligible senescence provided biologists with a conundrum: How better reproductive success accompanies age among some species. Such observations made an overall unifying theory that explains aging less likely. Science always incorporates a search for nomothetic—singular laws—that govern observations. In fact, the primary aim of all science is to observe, describe and predict. The great optimism of the mid-1800s followed by the resurgence of scientific knowledge in the 1900s further promoted this search for an underlying pattern. Biology was the first contender for a unifying theory of aging.

Biology of Aging

One of the few all-encompassing laws in biology, determined in turn by physics, is Kleiber's Law. After the second World War, Max Klieber, a Swiss agricultural chemist, predicted that mass determines metabolism, and metabolism determines longevity. Across species, larger animals with slower metabolism live longer. Metabolism is the body engine, and the observation was that the faster our biological operating speed, the shorter our life. Larger animals tend to live longer and have lower metabolism. This theory has been elaborated in 2000 with a study on nearly 4,100 longevity records for a variety of fish, reptile, amphibian, bird, and mammalian species including humans. Four primary findings resulted. First, longevity is positively correlated with body size between orders; a large species lives longer, but within species, being small is not necessarily detrimental. Secondly, animals that fly (i.e. birds and bats), are armored (turtles; armadillos) or live underground (moles; mole rats) tend to live longer than what is predicted from body size alone. Third, lifespans vary tremendously within species, with some animals living 50 times longer than others. Body size, metabolic rate, and brain size all positively correlate with life span. Fourth, primates comprise an exception. As long-lived mammals, the great apes (i.e. gorillas; chimpanzees) are long-lived primates, and humans consist of extraordinarily long-lived great apes; human longevity exceeds nearly all other species, both relatively and absolutely. This system places longevity in a very biologically constrained form. Our genetic and evolutionary makeup seems to determine our longevity. Such a beautiful single theory—nomothetic approach—to longevity had a good run, but it came across some problems and anomalies.

Kleiber's Law was complicated by Caleb Finch's "negligible senescence." The outliers that Finch exposed not only did not conform to the lifespan predicted, but these species showed no observable age-related increases in mortality rate, no decreases in reproduction rate after maturity, and no observable age-related decline in physiological capacity or disease resistance. It seems that although a general rule exists that determines the lifespan of most species, some exceptions endure. The American physician, poet, professor, lecturer, and author Oliver Wendell Holmes, Sr. said it best: "The young man knows the rules, but the old man knows the exceptions." If we were searching for exceptions where would we start looking?

The Geneticists

Simple experiments in the late 1970s and 80s changed all this dramatically. The three seminal research studies all have one thing in common—how the body preserves energy through growth hormones. If nature can manipulate longevity, surely all we need to do is to find the mechanism so that we can copy it.

A classic experiment by Michael Rose began manipulating the life spans of fruit flies by allowing them to reproduce only at late ages. The subsequent progeny of flies evolved longer life spans and greater reproduction over the next dozen generations. If our parents delayed producing us, then, our body seems to know to conserve energy in order to live longer. Nature allows future generations to pass on their genes at later periods in their life, and in order to do this, giving them longer life.

The second type of experiment uses examples from nature, which were emulated in the laboratory at U.C San Francisco by Cynthia Kenyon. Kenyon noticed that a naturally occurring disorder in some flatworms resulted in them living much longer than their peers. Through a series of trials in eliminating individual genes, the research team managed to chemically knock-out the gene daf-2 which partially disables receptors that are sensitive to two hormones—insulin and a growth hormone called IGF-1. This experiment nearly doubled the flatworms' lifespans. These long-lived worms looked and acted younger than their control group, implying that extending the lifespan also extends healthy life. By conserving energy, weakening insulin and a growth hormone, the flatworms lived longer.

Richard Miller and his infamous mouse called Yoda (now deceased) contributed to the third type of genetic observation on aging. Again, nature led the way in showing the longevity advantage of having less growth hormone. Like other dwarf mice, Yoda had a natural genetic mutation that obstructs the production of growth and thyroid hormones. Dwarf mice tend to grow to only about a third the size of normal mice, which helps them live about 40 percent longer. Three types of mice share this longevity characteristic—Snell, Ames and Laron dwarf mice. Even though these mice produce growth hormone, it is still growth-restricted because it is unable to respond to the hormone. The common denominator is that these mice have stunted growth—through either their lack of production or lack of sensitivity to growth hormone—that correlates with increased lifespan. Alternatively, these experiments have emboldened scientists to argue that a death clock seems to exist that can be modified by manipulating genes involved in someway with growth hormones—likely to be more than one gene—and secondly, that longevity is associated with being healthy. But other interpretations exist. Surprisingly, two inclusive and complimentary theories both explain these findings.

Antagonistic Pleiotropy and Disposable Soma

The theory of Antagonistic Pleiotropy suggests that some genes have contradictory effects at different ages. Genes which might enhance one's reproductive success at a younger period—e.g., genes that increase testosterone in men, resulting in more muscle mass and masculine secondary sexual characteristics—may at an older age have detrimental effects on long-term survival. In the testosterone example, a key later-life effect is the elevated risk of cancer.

Natural selection tends to favor these kinds of genes because they maximize fitness and reproduction (the passing of genes) at a younger age, while higher mortality occurs in post-reproduction stage and therefore have little impact on increasing numbers of offspring. The second theory, Disposable Soma, states that given finite resources to maintain and repair cells and organs, the body conserves energy and protects itself just long enough to pass on its genes. The body is maintained long enough to enable it to pass on its genes. The two theories operate complementarily.

In all genetic studies—whether involving manipulation or observation in nature—extended lifespan correlates with stunted growth or late life progeny. Does delayed growth stamp an expiration date onto our genes? If we are stunted in growth, or our parents were older when producing us, our bodies seem to know that they need to live longer in order to pass on our genes. The genes are the same, but they have been imprinted with an expiration date and allow the organism to life longer, a process that we don't yet fully understand. As with all genetic work, many confounders exist. How genes come to be expressed in the real world is not a simple process. There is no direct translation from the genotype—the genes—to the phenotype—how they get to be expressed in nature. We might have genes that predispose us to acquire a certain disease (for example diabetes), but perhaps through better diet we might not express this predisposition. The environment can intervene, as in the case of epigenetics— the ability for some conditions, such as diet, exercise, environmental conditions to switch on or off some specific genes—demonstrates conclusively. Even if we accept that stunted growth might preserve energy and improve lifespan, other genetic, health, or environmental factors might negate such gains.

Such is the case in south Ecuador, where a group of more than 250 individuals have Laron syndrome—IGF-1 deficiency. Similar to Richard Miller's mouse Yoda, who had a deficiency in a gene responsible for this primary growth hormone. This genetic condition affected humans to grow to less than four feet tall. As also found in mice, this stunted growth appears to protect Laron patients from developing cancer. However, the apparent protection does not translate to longer lifespans, as this Ecuadorian group is inflicted by self inflicted physical trauma and alcoholism. A schism exists between lifespan and theoretical lifespan, related to human behavior.

Human behavior, unlike that of mice, fruit flies or flatworms, is more complex. Such behavior—alcohol, smoking, risk behaviors—have a direct impact on lifespan. Sometimes our genes, or how we manipulate their expression, change our behavior, which in turn extends our life. This is the story of Eunuchs and the search for a switch that extends longevity in humans.

Eunuchs

Historically, and as recently as the 19th century, eunuchs were common across the world. Castrati boys— castrated before puberty—were among the most esteemed singers especially in Catholic churches in Italy. By banning women from singing in churches, castrati were prized. At its peak, 5,000 castrati—comprised of 8-year old boys— castrated to preserve their unbroken voices. The Sistine Chapel retained the last of the castrati singers in 1913. His name was Alessandro Moreschi, who died in 1922 at the age of 64. However, some historians suspect that Domenico Mancini, who sang in the papal choir until 1959, was a secret castrato. A recording exists of an interview he participated in when he was 31 years of age, where we get a glimpse into his eerily melodic singing. Most had prized careers in the opera houses in Europe. Elsewhere, eunuchs served as hired staff in harems and imperial palaces in China, Korea, Japan, the rest of Asia and the Middle East, as well as in Europe and Russia.

In the 18th century members of a Christian sect called the Skoptzy, also called the White Doves—in order to attain their ideal sanctity subjected themselves to castration, despite the bible saying nothing about cutting one's testicles off. They believed that the Messiah would not come until the Skoptsy numbered 144,000 (Bible Rev. 14:1,4): "And I looked, and, lo, a Lamb stood on the mount Sion, and with him an hundred forty and four thousand, having his Father's name written in their foreheads...These are they which were not defiled with women; for they are virgins."

Further east, in China, eunuchs played a more central role in government. The emperor maintained approximately 2,000 in his service, while the imperial princes and princesses each had about 30, and various family members were allowed 10 or so eunuchs each. Although in this context castration was mostly a punishment, some subjected themselves to the procedure in order to gain employment. At the same time, during the Ottoman period, especially from the 16th century, black eunuchs from Ethiopia or Sudan were placed in charge of harems in the Ottoman court. Since Muslim religion prohibits castrations, Coptic priests castrated many of these boys at a monastery in Upper Egypt. The practice was pervasive and endemic.

In 1999, Jean Wilson and Claus Roehrborn investigated the long-term effects of castration. The effects included the enlargement of the pituitary gland, especially among those with an earlier castration. Skeletal changes included thinning of the bones of the skull and decreased bone mineral density. An increased incidence of fractures, however, does not appear to have been reported among the eunuchs. Some reported growth of breasts in the Ottoman court eunuchs, which is also evident in photographs of Skoptzy men and Chinese eunuchs. Shrinkage of the prostate was common among eunuchs—which is why female hormones are used to reduce prostate cancer in men. However, the authors could not resolve whether life spans differed in their study.

James Hamilton and Gordon Mestler with State University of New York conducted a study on life span difference earlier, in 1969. They studied the mortality of patients in a mental institution with a population of 735 intact White males, 883 intact White females, and 297 White eunuchs. As a result of the eugenics movement at the turn of the century, it was common practice to castrate mentally challenged children. Hamilton and Mestler reported that survival was significantly better among eunuchs than in intact males and females. This survival advantage started at age 25 years and continued throughout their lives. The life expectancy for eunuchs was 69.3 years compared to 55.7 years for intact males. Males castrated at 8-14 years of age— before sexual maturation—were longer lived than males castrated at 20-39 years of age—after sexual maturation. Castration reduced the age of death by 0.28 years for every year of castration from age 39 and younger.

In 2012 Kyung-Jin Min from the Inha University, and his Korean colleagues, supported this observation. In their study, the authors reported that during the Chosun Dynasty, between the 14th to early 20th centuries, Korean eunuchs lived 14 to 19 years longer than intact men. Researchers were able to identify 81 eunuchs, who were castrated as boys, and determined that they lived to an average age of 70, significantly longer than other men of similar social status. Three of the 81 eunuchs lived to 100. This is a centenarian rate that's far higher than would be expected today.

Many changes occur as a result of castration. The world was very different 600 years ago, or even 100 years ago. In most cases, it was a very violent environment where men suffered early mortality through wars, famine, and daily violent trauma. Eunuchs, because of their demeanor, might have escaped much of that onslaught of trauma. They might also have had more nurturing qualities that extended to caring for themselves better. We will never know. We do know that although castration had some physical consequences, reduced life expectancy was not one of them. The most obvious advantage of having testes, other than the ability to reproduce, is increased virility, muscle mass and energy. But such advantages need to be seen in context. The story of feeling good is more complex than simply an extract, a fountain of youth. The fact that all these studies focused on men remains shortsighted. With women across the world—without exception—living longer than men, a smart bet on longevity would favor women.

Even though some of the positive outcomes reported in these early studies have been criticized as a placebo effect, they were searching for something that was real: increased longevity. There remains much to learn and although we might find humor in a lot of the early experiments, they were useful in pushing the frontiers of science. With one eye on charlatans, we should keep the other eye on our future. Experimentation, despite its reliance on belief, a penchant for failure and being a lonely trek, remains a key way to learn about our amazing aging bodies.

Feeling good

We knew that testes contained the sperm that made conception possible, because castrated animals were no longer capable of breeding. Castration also pacified them. The same effects occur in men. The Cumming Manuscript Collection of the New York Academy of Medicine Library contains more than 1,200 references, abstracts, and documents concerning the early history of human castration. But the first debates about the relationship between longevity and eunuchs—boys and men who had their testicles and sometimes their penis removed surgically–took place in the early 1990s. Serge Abrahamovitch Voronoff (1866-1951), a French surgeon of Russian origin made the observation that eunuchs have a different lifespan. But like all observations, stereotypes and expectations existed beforehand.

Another earlier émigré, Charles Edouard Brown-Séquard (1817-18944), was a prolific and widely recognized scientist, having published more than 577 papers in his lifetime. Born on Mauritius he later moved to France, studying and gaining his medical degree. He devoted his later years to experimental medicine, in search of immortality. However, Brown-Séquard's impending infamy was not for immortality, but for an earlier observation he made related to spinal injury.

In 1850, Brown-Séquard identified a neurology syndrome that now carries his name. He noticed that damage to one half of the spinal cord resulted in paralysis and loss of sense of body on the same side as the injury, and a loss of pain and temperature sensation on the opposite side. These observations helped elucidate the sympathetic/parasympathetic nervous system in the spinal cord.

Back in Paris, he founded the *Journal de la physiologie de l'homme et des animaux*, which included one of his articles on the necessity of the adrenal glands to the continuance of life. In his later life, he was more and more dedicated to this work on longevity, looking at glands and their extracts. In 1889, at age 72, Brown-Séquard published a study in *The*

Lancet on the rejuvenating effects of self-administered extracts of dog and guinea pig testes.

Writing in the journal, he recalled that: "The day after the first subcutaneous injection, and still more after the two succeeding ones, a radical change took place in me . . . I had regained at least all the strength I possessed a good many years ago . . . My limbs, tested with a dynamometer, for a week before my trial and during the month following the first injection, showed a decided gain of strength . . . I have had a greater improvement with regard to the expulsion of fecal matters than in any other function . . . With regard to the facility of intellectual labour, which had diminished within the last few years, a return to my previous ordinary condition became quite manifest."

Feeling good is automatically associated with reversing aging. Brown-Séquard also reported that similarly dramatic benefits of extracts from rabbit and guinea pig testes had been observed in three men, aged 54, 56 and 68 years, whereas placebo injections of water in two other men had had no effect. Despite his claims for rejuvenation, Brown-Séquard died in 1894 at the age of 77. Maybe he did not find immortality, but he left behind a vision for experimentation with glands.

Although it is unlikely that by using Brown-Séquard's methods there would have been enough testosterone concentrations required for a biological effect, undeniably such experiments were the first published that showed positive outcomes of the use of "extracts."

Back to Serge Voronoff, his technique did not injecting himself with an "extract" like Brown-Séquard, but by grafting monkey testicle tissue into the scrotums of men. Being a student of Alexis Carrel (a Nobel Prize winner in medicine), Voronoff was adept at organ transplantation. He decided to use his transplantation skills to surgically implant slivers of monkey testicles into the scrotum of humans. He used monkeys because he saw how virile and strong they were—another reason could be that it is probably easier to harvest testicles from a monkey than a man. Results showed a dramatic effect. Publishing before/after pictures in esteemed journals of *Lancet* and *Scientific American*, Voronoff was able to show dramatic positive outcomes. By the Great Depression of the 1930s, over 500 men had received Voronoff's monkey balls therapy.

Voronoff reported many improvements: increased sex drive, better memory, the ability to work longer hours, better eyesight and a prolonged life. As if that was not enough, the great surgeon speculated that monkey balls therapy might be beneficial for people with 'dementia praecox' (premature dementia), which was later renamed by Emil Kraepelin, the father of Alzheimer's disease, as schizophrenia. It was no surprise therefore that this wonder therapy become very popular. In order to cope with the increasing demands, Voronoff set up his own monkey farm to harvest their testes, perched on the Italian Riviera. He also experimented with transplant practice on women. Although the general scientific community dismissed these results as a placebo or a hoax, the final scientific consensus at the time was that the grafts are more likely to be rejected by the body.

Despite Voronoff's medical competency, his reputation was marred by his association with the infamous American charlatan John Richard Brinkley (1885–1942). Brinkley—without a medical degree, but with a lot of business acumen—transplanted goat testicles into humans. He used goats because they appeared so virile—and again more accessible than monkeys or human testes. Operating a multitude of clinics and hospitals in several states, Brinkley promoted this procedure as a cure for a wide range of male ailments. In 1938, Morris Fishbein, the editor of the *Journal of the American Medical Association* and well known at the time as a debunker of quack medicine, attacked Brinkley by publishing a two-part series called *Modern Medical Charlatans.* In retaliation Brinkley took Fishbein to court for defamation and lost.

Other transplant copycats existed as well. The peak of testicle transplantation came with Paul Niehans (1882–1971), who claimed to have performed more than 50,000 "cellular therapy" treatments. Niehans' 1960 book *Introduction to Cellular Therapy*, addressing testicular secretions, again proved popular. He boasted celebrity patients that included Pope Pius XII, Bernard Baruch and Aristotle Onassis.

The idea that testes were important for rejuvenation also led to other experimentation with testes. Overlapping some of Voronoff's success, Eugen Steinach (1861–1944) in 1918 started performing the first vasectomies on humans for rejuvenation. Although sterilization—by cutting *vasa deferentia* from the testicles, had been around for some time and was a technique used on prisoners and mentally deficient people— by the turn of the 20th century the technique of vasectomy was being used to rejuvenate old men. Notable patients included Sigmund Freud and Nobel Prize poet William Butler Yeats. To this day, vasectomy does not appear to have resulted in any effect (good or bad) on health. These less competent experiments—although helping to build an edifice of the health benefits of testes—did not have the same prestige as Voronoff. But Voronoff, despite his scientific integrity, had his own personal nemesis.

David Hamilton, an experienced transplant surgeon, delivered the most public critique of Voronoff's legacy much later in his life through the publication of *The Monkey Gland Affair* in 1986. Hamilton discussed how animal tissue inserted into a human would not be absorbed, but would be instantly rejected. Hamilton jokes that at best, it would result in scar tissue, which might fool a person into believing the graft is still in place. This was seemingly the final death knell to Voronoff's legacy; that his procedure was inconsequential.

Many years passed until science caught up with Voronoff's genius. We have subsequently learned that sertoli cells, which surround testes, protect organs from being rejected. It is likely that the grafts did survive–so much so that modern organ transplantation techniques cover harvested organs with sertoli cells, collected from testes, to suppress the body from rejecting the transplant.

Although both Voronoff and his predecessor/mentor Brown-Séquard were ridiculed and vilified at the time, our currently better understanding of the endocrine system has resulted in increased validity to some of their claims. Experimentation, despite its frequent reliance on belief, serves as an essential learning tool in understanding our aging bodies. Although these early experiments lead to the development of endocrinology and to the recognition of testosterone and other hormones in the body, earlier experiments have been discounted and subsequently ignored. To this day, testosterone and aging still have an ambivalent relationship.

These experiments were continued in 1927 by a University of Chicago professor Fred Koch, and his student, Lemuel McGee. Koch extracted half a teaspoon of extract from a supply of 40 pounds of bull testes from the Chicago stockyards. By injecting this extract into a castrated chicken—a capon—he was able to show the revival of male characteristics. By 1935, the Dutch Kàroly Gyula David and his colleagues were able to identify the critical ingredient in testes—testosterone. This opened the door to the Nobel Prize in chemistry in 1939 to be given jointly to Adolf Friedrich Johann Butenandt "for his work on sex hormones" and Leopold Ruzicka "for his work on polymethylenes and higher terpenes". Basically, they partially synthesized testosterone. More importantly the Nobel Prize in chemistry baptized the field of endocrinology and the crazy men who experimented with extracts were no longer seen as crazy.

In 2010, Spanish physician Mercè Fernández-Balsells and her colleagues published a review of 51 studies of testosterone in older men. None of the studies reported any significant effect on mortality, prostate or cardiovascular outcomes. While earlier reviews reported negative prostate and cardiovascular events, ongoing research remains too vague to ascertain any causality. By 2016 the pendulum started swinging back the other way.

After initial unsuccessful trials, a clinical trial conducted in 2016 by Peter Snyder from the Perelman School of Medicine at the University of Pennsylvania, Philadelphia, and colleagues, reported that testosterone therapy in select older men with low levels of testosterone improved sexual function, improved walking ability and provided more vitality to the men. Sounding more like Brown-Séquard's 1889 paper in the *Lancet*. In other studies, improvement was negated by an increase in cancer and cardiovascular complications, complications that were selected out of this group of men in the Snyder study.

It seems that Brown-Séquard and Voronoff have been vindicated. After a century of research, we now know a lot more about the effects of testosterone. It is not a secret mechanism that promotes longevity. But once researchers got a taste of this claimed elixir of life, the search for that secret switch that turns off death has only grown.

Conclusion of Immortality All Around Us

Numerous organisms and cells in our bodies will continue to exist after we are gone. Animals exist that have the capacity to stay around forever. Nature knows no limits in its capacity to assign immortality. Our lifespans often seem to be predestined. Scientists have been looking at the switch that allows lifespan limitations to be switched off. The most likely host for the longevity switch is in our genes. Three seminal studies have succeeded in increasing longevity. Two involve the reduction in the production or utilization of growth hormone. The third study–that breeds eggs from older flies successfully increase longevity remains a mystery.

The effects of growth hormone are fairly straightforward to explain. The less fuel that goes into the body, the less stress exists on the body to grow. No one wants to be a stunted, barren adult, but some men had no choice in the past. Castrati and eunuchs have their stories to contribute to our knowledge of living longer. It seems that having less testosterone bodes well for long-term survivability. This differs from earlier studies of increasing testosterone making older men feel better. Feeling better might not necessarily mean living longer. The answer might be more elusive, even though nature keeps showing us how easy it is to create immortality.

So far, we have failed to simplify the issue of longevity. Genetics, by itself does not provide a complete answer. Although genetics does play a role in longevity, other factors moderate and modulate the effect of genes. Longevity is not determined by a single gene but is part of a survival package. It seems that genetics alone holds very little predictive power in explaining behavior. Once we leave the tidy confines of genetic studies, then the arguments start sounding more sociological. Genetic studies do not explain longevity despite the obvious fact that genetics relates to the variance we find across animals. Perhaps we are asking the wrong question. Instead of asking how to achieve immortality—which we have been pursuing since the dawn of humanity—perhaps we should ask: why did nature make us mortal?

∞

Chapter 2

Why Are We Mortal?

Eating, drinking, dying - three primary manifestations of the universal and impersonal life. Animals live that impersonal and universal life without knowing its nature. Ordinary people know its nature but don't live it and, if they think seriously about it, refuse to accept it. An enlightened person knows it, lives it, and accepts it completely. He eats, he drinks, and in due course he dies - but he eats with a difference, drinks with a difference, dies with a difference."

— Aldous Huxley (1962). *Island* New York. Harper & Row, (Page 242)

Evolutionary biologists see death as necessary for the species but detrimental to the individual. For a species to develop, a turnover must occur. Death results in genetic improvement in the next generation. The belief that genetics determines lifespan is not contested. A butterfly has a consistently shorter lifespan than a human. It is how genes influence death that attracts our attention. As discussed in Chapter 1, scientists have been looking for that elusive switch that will turn off death. All animals have a pre-determined maximum longevity. This is their lifespan. We accept that some animals live a certain amount of time, and we witness this every day. The most persuasive argument for the genetic influence on lifespan is that different animals have different lengths of life. Each species has a preordained life card. Although there might be variance within each species, consistency exists in the length of time a member of a species lives. How we make use of this maximum lifespan remains determined by our behavior. Enormous scientific and social interest exists in manipulating this expiration date. The study of genetics has been influenced by our "survival of the fittest" belief. Because earlier biologists did not recognize the benefits of aging, the survival of the fittest concept contends that aging escapes natural selection, and by so doing aging is therefore a mistake. But overall, the argument that eventually emerges from scientific literature is that aging is useful, and that it comprises part of the package of what make us human. That package is made possible by our genes. Without aging, our strategies for survival are diminished. Aging is, in fact, an integral component of the survival of the fittest.

Perhaps we can cheat nature to let us live longer. But we also know that lifespan doesn't respond like a timeswitch, predetermined and absolute. It is more of a suggested expiration date. What if we can manipulate conditions to extend this expiration date? Questions like this have motivated people from the earliest literature created by humankind, to the first philosophical musings, and later on to the emergence of science. The study of aging, and more accurately experimentation in aging, has spawned the disciplines of endocrinology, cryogenics, actuarial statistics and ingloriously, the whole industry related to "anti-aging."

Although many scientists have attempted to summarize the science of longevity across all species, I will focus nearly exclusively on humans. Although there are many variations in genetics that determines lifespan across species, we do not know the many different mechanisms. We need to explore how malleable this variance is, and what determines its elasticity. While most people die before age 75, others are increasingly celebrating their 100th birthday. The fastest growing group in our contemporary population is centenarians. What separates these people from the rest of the human population involves an intriguing journey of discovery and refutation of long held beliefs. To understand this variance, we must start with the first gerontological revolution among humans: the development of our bigger brain.

Bigger Brain, Longer Life

During 3.5 million years of human evolution, an enormous increase in brain size occurred. Other species did not show this incredible growth. It is purely a human phenomenon—from a brain volume of 300cm^3 found in Ramapithecuspunjabicus to the now extinct Homo neanderthalensis peak of 1460cm^3 falling back down to the modern homo sapiens of 1410 cm^3. Brain size is important for longevity. One traditional idea about the distinctions in brain size between humans' and other animals' stems from George Sacher's 1959 innovative analyses, correlating brain size with lifespan. Although some of his conjectures have been refined and some refuted in gerontology, the analyses remain robust. For humans, a larger brain translates to a longer life.

Table 1. Estimate of lifespan for hominids derived from fossil body weight and cranial capacity measurements.

		Time of Appearance (yr x 10^{-6})	Cranial Capacity (cm^3)	Lifespan (years)
1	Ramapithecuspunjabicus	14	300	42*
2	Australopithecus africanus	3	450	35-40
3	Australopithecus robustus	2.5	500	35
4	Australopithecus boisei	2	530	52*
5	Homo habilis	1.5	660	61*
6	Homo erectusjavanicus	0.7	860	40-60
7	Homo erectuspekinensis	0.25	1040	40-60
8	Homo europaeus pre-Wurm	0.1	1310	40-60
9	Homo neanderthalensis europaeus	0.045	1460	40-60
10	Homo sapiens europaeus Würm	0.015	1460	94*
11	Homo sapiens recent	0.01	1460	90
12	Homo sapiens modern (present)		1410	95

* Lifespan Predicted (against observed)

No skull has been recovered of the Denisovans (Altai) and therefore we do not have brain size estimates

Source: Modified from Table 2. Cutler, R. G. (1975).

Although Neanderthals were born with a similar size brain as modern humans, they seem to have exhibited a larger brain growth in adulthood. We do not know why, or the outcomes of this phenomenon. Much conjecture exists in our own limited understanding. Scientists try to understand observations by linking them in some causal fashion. Because Neanderthals became extinct, we assume that there was a "price" for their brain size. Referring to the Disposable Soma Theory and the Expensive Tissue hypothesis, the cost for having a larger brain might have resulted in their extinction. "The Neanderthal brain size growth phenotype suggests that brain size growth patterns imposed high metabolic costs." Steven Leigh with the University of Colorado, Boulder wrote in 2012 (page 596).

However, the Neanderthals did not become extinct, at least not completely. They passed on some of their genes to homo sapiens. They were not alone in passing their genes to modern humans.

In 2015, an international team of scientists led by Svante Pääbo, a geneticist at the Max Planck Institute working with the Russian scientist Anatoly Derevianko, found a tooth fossil in a cave in southern Siberia's Altai Mountains. The find–just one tooth—nevertheless yielded DNA from a vanished branch of our ancestors called the Denisovans. The emerging story is that both the Neanderthals and Denisovans emerged from Africa half a million years ago. As the Denisovans headed east, the Neanderthals spread westward, settling in the Near East and Europe. Some 50,000 years ago, they interbred with humans expanding from Africa along the coast of South Asia, contributing some of their DNA to modern humans. Although we now have three distinct branches of hominids intermixed within our modern bodies, we are likely to find many more genetic contributions with increasing knowledge of our ancient human diversity.

The turn of the 21st century saw the first results of the 1000 Genomes Project, studying genetic historical markers of human population. Before the discovery of the Denisovans, several studies detected Neanderthal ancestry in modern humans–suggesting that Neanderthal alleles may have helped modern humans to adapt to non-African environments, although we do not know that. These results show that the ancestral modern human gene pool—and the gene pools of Neanderthals, Denisovans (Altai) and other extinct hominins—were open systems that allowed exchange of genes among groups when they met. It is likely that other extinct hominins will be found in the near future and that their genetic traces will be found in modern humans. As of today, mainly Neanderthal genetic influence has been studied. Geneticists have looked at autosome and allosome chromosome, with allosome chromosome being the sex chromosome. Humans have a dual system of genes—diploid genome—that usually contains 22 pairs of clusters of genes, 46 chromosomes in total. The interbreeding of Neanderthals with modern humans introduced some genes (alleles) into modern humans. There must have been some advantages to this interchange, which worked for modern humans but apparently not for the Neanderthals. The distribution of this one variation of human gene can be seen in Table 2. Denisovans, on the other hand, have a different distribution.

Table 2: Genome-wide estimates of Neanderthal ancestry

	(%) X chromosomes	(%) autosomes
Han Chinese in Beijing, China	0.3	1.4
Han Chinese in South China	0.27	1.37
Japanese in Tokyo	0.26	1.38
Toscani in Italy	0.25	1.11
Iberian populations in Spain	0.23	1.07
Colombians in Medellin, Colombia	0.22	1.14
White Utah, USA	0.21	1.17
Mexican ancestry in Los Angeles	0.21	1.22
British England & Scotland	0.2	1.15
Puerto Ricans in Puerto Rico	0.2	1.05
Finnish in Finland	0.19	1.2
African ancestry in Southwest USA	0.07	0.34
African Luhya in Webuye, Kenya	0.04	0.08

Source: Adapted from Sankararaman, S., Hopf, H., Dix, I., & Jones, P. G. (2000). Table 1 (p.355).

For Denisovan genes the highest concentration of Denisovan geneses exists around Papua New Guinea,

Philippines, Eastern Indonesia, Australia and Near and Remote Oceania. Evidence suggests that the Denisovan genes are evident in Eastern Eurasian and Native American groups.

The lesson from these studies is that human development benefited from an intermixing of genes. It is likely that such contact—and we might not have even identified the extent of this contact—resulted in our brains growing. There are arguments that having too large a brain might be disadvantageous. When Gary Lynch and Richard Granger wrote about the Boskops skull in *Big Brain* in 2008, they caused a lot of controversy. The *Big Brain* refers to a new hominid found in South Africa with a cranial capacity of 1,980 cc, a third more than our modern human brain. Lynch and Granger argue that this translates to an IQ of 150, but we need to be cautious in over-generalizing. As with another find related to the Paracas elongated skulls in Peru and the Antarctic with maybe a cranial capacity 15%-25% larger than modern humans. There are serious methodological issues with the interpretations of these finds. But, with great caution, we have to ask whether having too big a brain might be a disadvantage. It could be too nutrient demanding, or it that having a great capacity to think can be psychologically disturbing. We can only conjecture. There could be a Goldilocks principle too, not too big, not too small but just right.

What remains perplexing is how a larger brain increases longevity. Many possible reasons exist, but if we stick with the genetic story, we have to admit that there must be some biological advantage.

In the history of science, the use of cranial capacity to measure brain size and then to extrapolate the findings to other personal characteristics had a darker side. In early attempts to classify people, the classification was based not just on the phenotype—how the individual looked—but also on the individual's assumed social, psychological and intellectual characteristics. This resulted in eugenics—a euphemism for racism, that you can discern intellectual and social characteristics from how a person looks. We still see remnants of eugenics in science today.

In terms of cranial capacity and brain size, the work of Samuel George Morton (1799–1851) stands out. Morton, a prolific experimentalist, showed how cranial capacity, and therefore brain size, differed between "races" of modern humans. Such observations engendered the idea that humans with different physiological characteristics have different intelligence. Eugenics, the belief that our biology determines our psychological and intellectual characteristics, is applied to "prove" the inferiority of certain groups to others. It took more than a century for a valid critique of these studies to emerge. In 1981, Harvard University professor Stephen Jay Gould published *The Mismeasure of Man,* dispelling the accuracy of these early studies. Gould argued that in most cases the researcher unintentionally biased the results. Bird seeds, and later lead shot pellets, were packed into the cranium at variable degrees of compaction. Although Gould's findings and conclusion resulted in widespread refutation—a furor of vitriolic backlash from psychologists, statisticians, and microbiologists, among others—it remains unlikely that we will ever dispel the idea that a bigger brain translates to greater intelligence. A bigger brain with greater longevity might, however, provide a less contested association.

Most would ask why a larger brain results in longer life? But that is the wrong question to ask. The biological question to ask is the obverse of this. Why does genetic survival require longer life through a larger brain? For the answer to this question we must turn again to biologists. If life was simply a game of transferring genes, like in a relay race, where after you pass on your baton you can relax and have a martini–then living longer after the act of passing on your baton has no biological value. In that context—life being a relay race—genetics should not determine longevity. But the reality is different. The social aspect of genetics should not be overlooked. In reality, humans not only transfer genes, but also culture, nurturing environment, a tribe, language, a built environment, and political context. This is what attracts us to our partners. The theory of population survival dictates that one of these attributes includes having a bigger brain in order to store information to impart to the next generation, and a sufficient life expectancy to be able to impart that information.

Other animals have developed a similar strategy for survival: having fewer offspring but investing more into their nurturing. As adopted by humans, this strategy is referred to as K-selection species. "K" is the symbol used to define the carrying capacity—how large a population the environment can support—coined by the ecologists Robert MacArthur and Edward Wilson to differentiate how species differ in their survival strategies. In 1967, the authors formulated *The Theory of Island Biogeography*. Within this species-specific strategy, they argue for an alternate method for survival–to have a higher turnover (death rate). This method involves having a lot of children in the hope that a few will survive and pass on their genes. The "r" refers to the statistical symbol for rate of growth, the alternative biological strategy to "K."

Biologists deal effectively with longevity. They categorize species based on whether they are long-lived or short-lived. Each species has a different strategy for survival: Have many children and live short lives, or invest in fewer children and live longer. Mathematical models show that whichever strategy is followed, species efficient in both strategies showed similar results–adaptability and therefore survival of the genes.   Both r and K strategies could be effective for a particular species. Nature has selected species that are good at both types of strategies. These strategies also have mythological names: *Semelparity* refers to "r" strategists, and *Iteroparity* for "K" strategists.

"r" and "K" Populations

The shotgun approach to survival strategy is known as *Semelparous*. To produce many offspring and then die, leaving them to fend for themselves. The name comes from a mythological story of Semele. Many different variants of this story exist, all of which share the same core meaning. In Greek mythology, the god of thunder, Zeus, fell in love with one of his priestesses, the mortal Semele. She was accustomed to swimming naked in the river Asopus to cleanse herself of the sacrificial bull's blood. There, disguised as an eagle, the voyeur Zeus fell in love with her and eventually consummated his love eventually resulting in Semele becoming pregnant. Zeus' wife, the goddess Hera, jealous of this new love, disguised herself as an old disagreeable woman—a crone—and befriended Semele. In a display of bravura Semele confided in Hera that her lover was the god Zeus, Hera's husband. Hera pretended not to believe her and questioned her story, telling Semele that she must be mistaken, as she had never seen him for the god that he is. Hera knew that exposing himself as a god, Zeus in all his mighty energy, will burn Semele into ashes. In order to prove to the crone that she was right, Semele asked Zeus to give her one thing that she asks. Eager to please her, Zeus agreed. When she asked him to reveal himself in all his divine glory he realized that mortals cannot look upon him without burning. Despite his protestations, he unmasked himself and in his lightning brilliance consumed Semele in a fiery blaze. Zeus however quickly rescued the fetus from her womb, sewing it into his thigh where a few months later, Dionysus was born.

Semele always refers to death after reproduction. The word *parous* is from the Greek meaning to reproduce. So *Semelparous* describes a single reproductive episode before death. This very specific strategy consists of investing everything in one last ditch at reproduction before death engulfs you. Unlike Zeus, however, this strategy requires multiple simultaneous births. The best example of this exists as spawning Pacific salmon. In most cases, both male and females suffer the same fate. Among the Australian *Antechinus stuartii*, brown marsupials, all males die shortly after mating in their 11th or 12th month of life at the same time each year. They are the smallest semelparous mammal. They die from environmental conditions that they bring onto themselves. Increased physiological stress from the period of breeding, seasonal aggression and competition triggers increased stress levels, which then cause the suppression of the immune system. After the collapse of their immune system, the animal dies from blood and intestinal parasites, and from liver infections. In addition, in the wild, many females similarly die after rearing their first litter, although some do survive a second year. *Antechinus stuartii* "reproduce" themselves to death.

In contrast, the other survival strategy is that of a sniper approach, known as *Iteroparous*. The word *iter* is from the Greek meaning to pass by or repeat, and *pario*, to reproduce. *Iteraparous* is devoid of a colorful mythological story. Examples of *iteroparous* animals are cows, humans, many insects, many bird species, and primates. This strategy is to have few offspring but to invest in their nurturing.

The simplicity of the concept of r and K strategies allows us to quickly differentiate very different species on the basis of their strategy to pass on their genes. Organisms in hazardous environments will maximize reproduction and thus be r-selected while organisms in non-hazardous environments will maximize their performance under crowded conditions and thus be K-selected. Therefore, r-selection will favor rapid development, small body size, and a short lifespan while K-selection will favor delayed development, larger body size, and a longer lifespan. Nature allows many types of survival strategies along this continuum.

Longevity in this case is becomes part of the "genetic" package because it allows for long-term nurturing of offspring. In this case, we can understand how lifespan becomes a biological pawn in the strategies for survival. Although "strategy" implies a conscious decision, in this case strategy is more on the part of nature giving advantage to this attribute. A longer lifespan, from a biological standpoint, comes with the survival package. Our longevity is an integral part of what makes us K-strategists. For instance, humans, whales, or elephants are K-selected while mice and voles are r-selected. If we consider the wide range of lifespans among animals (including mammals), as well as factors correlating with longevity, r and K selection provides a useful model for understanding such variation among different populations. Our longevity is part of a biological package, necessary for the population to survive—which firmly identifies humans as social survivalists. As part of this K-population strategy, we need a big brain to enable us to accumulate experiences and transmit wisdom to emerging generations.

Having a bigger brain plays into the story of an evolving K-population strategy. With a larger brain, humans found the necessary time–our longevity–to enable us to transfer knowledge. Without increased longevity, having a bigger brain is useless. It's like having a powerful computer without software. Longevity allows us to download the software. Longevity is needed for our survival. The ability to live long enough to nurture younger cohorts is part of hat makes humans so successful as a species. This is a very different story from the survival of the fittest narrative which narrowly focus on genes alone. These are social, intergenerational transfers. The narrative fits better when discussing a group or community rather than an individual. Given that humans have one of the largest brains among mammals, are we perhaps too successful at surviving. Are we so good at controlling our environment, protecting our progeny that we might be prone to overbreeding?

Are Humans Overbreeding?

In the late 1700s a new narrative was gaining ground among philosophers. Is society heading in the right direction? During this period of Enlightenment (1685-1815), a paradigm shift took place in science, philosophy, society and politics–which culminated in the French Revolution. By replacing the French monarchy, nobility, and political elite with a political and social order based on human reason with freedom and equality for all, Europe ushered in a period of social and scientific introspection.

To answer some of these questions, philosophers and scientists took to mathematics, the language of god. The mathematics of populations was initiated with Leonhard Euler, followed by Johann-Heinrich Lambert in the late 1700s. Both developed a mathematical law of death using data on human mortality from London (1753–1758) that had very accurate data. Two diametrically opposed views emerged. One view held a dystopian view while the other held a utopian view of population growth.

On the utopian side, the writings of William Godwin, Marquis de Condorcet, David Hartley and Joseph Priestley emphasized the power of our intellect and proposed that overpopulation was the result of social conditions and not innate, biological determinism. They especially pointed out that inequities in wealth and property cause the ills of society rather than population itself. William Godwin goes much further with a controversial claim—which he later redacted—that in a perfect society, humans would attain earthly immortality as a matter of natural development. "For if the mind could gain power over all other matter", Godwin asks, then "why not over the matter of our own bodies?"

Such luminaries as David Hume, Robert Wallace, Adam Smith, and Richard Price on the other hand championed the dystopian view. Robert Wallace a minister in the Church of Scotland, argued that population growth could weaken prosperity. Wallace conjectured that even under a perfect government where "poverty, idleness, and war [would be] banished; the earth made a paradise; universal friendship and concord established, and human society rendered flourishing in all respects," such a world will collapse "not by the vices of men, or their abuse of liberty, but by the order of nature itself." Overpopulation. We will become overly successful at reproducing.

The blight of civilization is overpopulation, which will destroy any possibility of a utopian outcome. In his writings, Wallace conjectured that slowing population growth would require "cruel and unnatural customs." But this and other reservations did not stop the most powerful seismic shock in social philosophy at the time–the rise of the Malthusian revolution. The Malthusian argument transformed how we thought about human populations. Reverberations of which can still be felt today.

Between 1798 and 1826, the English Anglican cleric Thomas Malthus published six editions of *An Essay on the Principle of Population*, arguing that populations grow logarithmically (doubling every 50 years or so) and food production increased linearly (increasing by numerical stages). With such simple assumptions, it was easy to see that at some point, populations will outpace food production. This erroneous observation resulted in a single conclusion—a fairly simple and resilient conclusion—that populations will eventually outstrip their food supply. The problem, therefore, is that populations are growing faster than we can feed them. Our behavior conflicts with our own capacity to survive. But these mathematical assumptions can also go the opposite way.

Population might grow exponentially, but it also decreases exponentially. This is the reality that we are seeing today. Population decline has occurred across all industrialized countries over the past five decades. Even in Africa, with the highest fertility rate on earth, a precipitous decline in birth rate exists. Without children populations will not grow, and every country in the World, including Nigeria, are seeing a decline in the number of children women are having.

In addition, food supply can grow exponentially, not just incrementally. No law slows the general production of food, as the USA has shown by advancing industrial agricultural technology. At the time, the Malthusian revolution was useful because it promoted a belief in the survival of the individual rather than the survival of a group or community. Everyone was out for himself. The K-strategists were in it for themselves.

Gomperts-Makeham Law

These early discussions highlight the worldwide conflict that existed. There was, and remain a perception that life is characterized by a struggle to survive. By 1825, Benjamin Gompertz developed a formula that mapped the probability of mortality across age. He found that populations followed a sigmoid function, with a broad, elongated "S" shaped curve on its side. Populations start to grow slowly, then reach a peak efficiency before they start to decline in growth. For mortality, the concluding part of this curve, Gompertz charted the probability of dying due to diminished resilience as a result of age. His formula was that mortality rate doubled every eight years for people over 30 years of age. Among humans, there were two exceptions—very young children and very old adults. This mortality rate was defined as increasing vulnerability to mortality. The older you are the more likely that you will die. This formula was improved by the addition of a universal death threat, regardless of age, which was introduced by William Matthew Makeham in 1860. This constant reflects the continuous exposure to disease—which varies according to environment or geography. In combination, the Gomperts-Makeham law represents an accurate probability of dying, across ages and differing conditions.

It seems that by the middle of the 1800s, a clear understanding of the harsh conditions for survival was becoming widely accepted. The social reality at the time must have been violent and impoverished. Recorded instances existed where this struggle exposed itself in disturbing fashion. Charles Darwin, while travelling with his grandfather Erasmus Darwin—a contemporary of Malthus—was attacked in his carriage by a group of destitute people. The idea of a struggle for survival must have influenced Darwin to adopt the concept of struggle to formulate a new biological theory. With the subtitle of his 1859 *Origin of the Species* "Preservation of Favoured Races in the Struggle for Life," Darwin successfully discounted more than a century of scientific thought on the survival of the fittest. The concept, survival of the fittest, caught the feeling of the century despite Darwin never using this phrase himself.

Darwinian Aging

In his writing, Darwin does not refer to aging. Although he might have seen aging as related to inherited characteristics, he never developed this idea further: "I have stated . . . that there is some evidence to render it probable, that at whatever age any variation first appears in the parent, it tends to reappear at a corresponding age in the offspring." Darwin's fundamental thesis was that life is a struggle for survival. This was a radically new idea in biology. Due to the relentless pressure of population growth, this struggle for life dictated that those that adapt to the environment have a better chance of survival. But if aging does not promote procreation, how can it promote survival of the population? Within a K-population strategy, what component does aging contribute, if any?

This conceptual vacuum left the role of aging open to two possible interpretations. The first was that aging only benefits the individual and has no evolutionary attribute. The second argument is that aging allows for the group to benefit in some way. The argument that aging has no evolutionary benefit has dominated scientific views for more than two centuries. Although Darwin did not address this, Alfred Russel Wallace filled the vacuum. Wallace, a contemporary of Darwin and co-discoverer of natural selection, argued that aging is "programmed death" and benefits the group when people die. He wrote that "...when one or more individuals have provided a sufficient number of successors they themselves, as consumers of nourishment in a constantly increasing degree, are an injury to those successors. Natural selection therefore weeds them out." (p.23). As long as they have already reproduced, older people are not only useless; they are a liability since they consume our limited resources. Nature will benefit from the removal of older adults—and here we have an exact age, those past reproductive capability. You are old once you have reproduced.

This concept, that from an evolutionary perspective aging is useless, was later reaffirmed in a lecture entitled 'The duration of life' in 1881, by the German biologist August Weismann. Initially, imitating Wallace, Weismann argued that aging—becoming frail and then dying—although detrimental to the individual, helps the species by removing older members from depleting limited food supplies. Later he changed this "injuriousness" interpretation of old age and merely considered old age as neutral for the biological species: "It is of no importance to the species whether the individual lives longer or shorter, but it is of importance that the individual should be enabled to do its work towards the maintenance of the species..." We can see how deeply the philosophy envisioning a limited amount of resources—propounded by Malthus and enshrined in Darwin's theory of "favoured Races"—continued to inspire modern thought.

Weismann, responding to his predecessor William Godwin, saw immortality as futile in terms of our evolutionary biology. As long as we reproduce, nature does not care whether you live forever or die immediately after reproducing. His theory of *panmixia* predicted that characteristics that do not promote reproduction— specifically mentioning the possibility of immortality—will eventually disappear. Immortality has no benefits for evolution. According to Weisman, if we take *panmixia* to the extreme, ideally nature will ensure that we will live just long enough to reproduce. *Panmixia* predicts that aging will be bred out of our populations. But aging was not being "bred out." If anything, aging was increasing.

With the discovery of genetics, evolutionary biology assumed a more focused and negative interpretation of aging. When John Burdon Sanderson Haldane (1892–1964) published *New Paths in Genetics* in 1941, he further argued that aging is immaterial to natural selection—it is just an artifact. A critical factor to this interpretation was the existence of Huntington's disease, a debilitating inherited disease that mimics Amyotrophic Lateral Sclerosis (also known as ALS, Lou Gehrig's disease), Parkinson's and Alzheimer's disease simultaneously. Since the disease emerges late in life, on average at age 35.5 years, Haldane argued that natural selection has no effect on weeding it out. As with Huntington's disease, aging is not a player in natural selection because it is expressed after the cards are dealt. This result in what Peter Medawar (1915–1987) called "mutation accumulation." Natural selection allows any negative characteristic in old age to collect since it cannot select out these characteristics at the time reproduction occurs. Aging becomes the genetic dustbin of humanity.

What cannot be weeded out remains hidden in a genetic time bomb that becomes apparent as we age. Not only is aging a terminal refuse dump of bad genes, but there might be positive traits that are selected for early in life that turn out to be lemons in old age. This argument, made by the American George C. Williams (1926), noted that natural selection favors genes that would be beneficial in youth but which might later result in deleterious aging characteristics— Michael Rose in 1982, would later name this idea "antagonistic pleiotropy."

Aging as a Genetic Dustbin

Antagonistic Pleiotropy was first proposed by George C. Williams in 1957 to specifically explain aging. Pleiotropy is the phenomenon where one or a few genes control more than one trait. The antagonism part comes from the negative effect that emerges later. For example, testosterone in men might result in an attractive muscular body in youth, masculine features such as a deep voice and facial hair (pleiotropy), but it also increases the likelihood of prostate cancer in older age–hence the antagonistic part of pleiotropy. Since the positive aspects of the pleiotropic gene are promoted through natural selection, the antagonistic aspect (prostate cancer) sneaks into the gene pool. Prostate cancer develops mainly in older men. Today one man in seven will be diagnosed with prostate cancer during his lifetime. The average age at the time of diagnosis is about 66 and is very rare before the age of 40.

Aging is seen as an invisible cloak that sneaks bad genes into the gene pool by hiding them under positive traits when young. Aging, in this view, has subverted the whole process of natural selection by disguising itself as a positive attribute in early life and then transforming—in a Jekyll and Hyde metamorphosis—into a liability. Somehow nature has been hoodwinked into allowing people to get old. But how can nature be so naive? The answer again comes from studying populations, this time by applying mathematical modeling to population survival success.

Package for Survival

With the increasing complexity of our understanding, philosophers (and later mathematicians) needed to incorporate more than the individual characteristic, or one community in their approach. Mathematically looking at broader issues rather than then just death statistics can only make more accurate predictions.

The modern theory of the population dynamic started after the Age of Enlightenment with Alfred James Lotka (1880–1949), who formally introduced mathematical theory to biology. The Lotka–Volterra equation—developed at the same time but independently by Vito Volterra—are also known as the predator–prey equations. They describe the dynamics of biological systems in which two species interact, one as a predator and the other as prey. The Lotka–Volterra equation predict that at some point there will be a balance. The number of predators and prey will level off and reach equilibrium. Without prey, predators cannot survive.

That same year, in 1907, the Swedish statistician Axel Gustav Sundbarg concluded that a human population's predisposition to grow or decline is determined by its age structure. He explicitly stated that a population's state of civilization can be measured by its death rate. Aging might not make a genetic contribution but it has mathematical importance. Peter Medawar's observation supports this view that the influence of natural selection declines with age. But in mathematical models, age structure is important.

The seminal argument came in 1954 with Lamont C. Cole's paper on life history consequences for populations. With this paper, Cole argued for a closer application of mathematics to biology. Cole also moved the discussion from r- and K-strategies to a different level. This line of thought ushered in a more social interpretation of biology, which hauled aging with it.

Cole started his review by exposing the arrogance of some assumptions made in mathematical models, which biologists were reluctant to accept. While on the biology side, he also expressed his uncertainty in their models by identifying that the r- and K-strategies show great inter-variance—including longevity—which is not addressed. Cole describes survival strategies—defined as "reproductive capacities sufficient to replace the existing species population" (p. 104)—as a balance. His mathematical formula defined the optimum balance. A too-successful species can overrun their environment (Malthusian prediction). Too unsuccessful and they become extinct. Within this formula, the age of reproduction was found to be an important factor in determining the efficiency of the species. But such conjectures were based on a static lifespan that does not change. If you are expected to live to 60 years, then there must be an optimal age at which one must reproduce. In addition, Cole acknowledged that there are many different strategies—life-history patterns—that can affect survival. "The number of conceivable life-history patterns is essentially infinite, if we judge by the possible combinations of the individual features that have been observed. Every existing pattern may be presumed to have survival values under certain environmental conditions…" (p.135).

Cole's overwhelming contribution to the debate is the knowledge that population survival is based on a balance across an infinite number of potential variables. His extensive mathematical models concluded that every existing pattern has some survival value under certain environmental conditions. There is no perfect strategy because the environment changes. Cole's conclusion that although the possible life-histories are essentially infinite, they are as important as anything else in our survival. Some life histories include: Age at first reproductive event, aging, and the number and size of offspring. "Comparative studies of life histories appear to be fully as meaningful as studies of comparative morphology, comparative psychology, or comparative physiology" (p. 134-135).

Genetics of aging theories, relying on mathematical models, have concluded that many factors can comprise a "package" for survival. Characteristics that are psychological, anatomical and physiological are as important as genetic characteristics. As a result of these broader definitions, evolutionary biology became more social. Moving away from seeing evolutionary biology—and therefore aging—as a genetic dustbin, to viewing aging and longevity as part of a social package transformed the concept of natural selection. The move is from a purely individual and selfish strategy to a strategy that includes the interests of the group, the family and the kin. Kin, family and community are interchangeable in definition.

To study the importance of family, William Hamilton (1936–2000) went back to basics, applying Malthusian dynamics as a measure of fitness for a population with overlapping generations. The model of Kin Selection proposes that fitness or beneficial genes include both those held by the individual as well as those held by their family. Accordingly, a particular behavior is favored by natural selection if it increases an individual's survival. This model—which later benefited from the mathematical models developed by Brian Charlesworth—produced accurate predictive outcomes. Unlike earlier evolutionary biologists who assumed that evolution was similar to a relay race where the baton—in this case the genes—are passed from one generation to another, Hamilton suggested an overlap among generations, where the older generations influence younger generations. The ultimate test of this kin selection hypothesis came with the development of evolutionary game theory.

Evolutionary Game Theory

By 1973 John Maynard Smith and George Price introduced evolutionary game theory to the kin selection model. While classic game theory requires players making rational choices on the basis of their individual gains, evolutionary game theory is based on acknowledging what others might do as well. The key insight of evolutionary game theory is that many decisions are dependent upon what others might do. Maynard Smith argued that evolution does not benefit individuals (since everyone dies), rather that evolution is designed to benefit the species (or the community). The strategy that humans employ is based on benefits to the species rather than benefits solely to the individual. This insight was revolutionary. It transformed the argument from one where aging is a genetic dustbin, to one where aging becomes part of a package and where older adults contribute, in as yet unknown ways, to the survival of a population.

Following this insight in 2002, 51 scientists including some of the most respected scientists such as Jay Orshansky and Leonard Hayflick, published a position statement in *Scientific American* stating that "…longevity determination is under genetic control only indirectly" and "… aging is a product of evolutionary neglect, not evolutionary intent." Again, aging is not seen as a contributing part of the package of K-strategies, but rather as an unintentional enigma. As we have seen, in terms of human survival, this assumption is not correct.

Having grandparents who can babysit, provide support to parents and grandkids and provide a safe and nurturing environment can–and does–have positive effects on the "kin," the family as a whole and the community at large. These social benefits occur in addition to the transfer of capital that older adults accumulate and pass on, both during their lifetime and after they die. These are social influences, occurring in an environment that is also biological. Social influences play a role in evolutionary biology.

George Christopher Williams at Stony Brook University used this same argument, that there is a family advantage to older age in explaining menopause. Williams argued that menopause allows older women to minimize mortality through childbirth and to redirect their efforts by supporting existing offspring, promotes the "Grandmother Hypothesis." A grandmother provides a documented beneficial effect on the reproductive success of her children and the survival of her grandchildren. Genetic (survival), economic (capital transfer) as well as social (protection) advantages accrue through long-lived grandparents. The components of evolutionary biology are therefore difficult to comprehend. Referring back to Cole's quote, "The number of conceivable life-history patterns is essentially infinite...."

Evolutional biology depends on certain fixed constants. Cole highlighted some of these, and much earlier, the Swedish statistician Axel Gustav Sundbarg, emphasized the importance of age in keeping population dynamics in balance. This suggests that as long as children are born and people die at the same rates, then equilibrium, a balance, exists. But this equilibrium is no longer evident in the world.

On one side, we see all industrialized countries in the world showing a decline in fertility rate—Total Fertility Rate (TFR), the number of children an average woman will have—to a level that will not replace the existing population. This has never happened before in human history. Developing countries are quickly following suit. Even Nigeria, the largest country in Africa, is showing TFR declines that have not occurred in many other countries, falling from 6.4 in 1955 (the average woman gave birth to about 6 children) to 6.1 in 2005 and 5.7 in 2016. By the next decade, Nigeria will see a TFR half of what it is today. And this slowing down is unlikely to change as we have seen in industrialized countries.

Industrialized countries have a TFR of less than 1.3 per woman. A Japanese survey in 2010 found that one in four unmarried men in their 30s are virgins. The figures are slightly less for women. Such a trend worries politicians, who have tried to cajole, incentivize, reward or otherwise implore women to have more children. But the die is cast, and women will continue to have fewer babies, and eventually populations will continue to shrink. Other than the short-term gain of allowing immigrants into a country, the ongoing population march is down a way-one street, heading toward negative population growth.

On the other side of the equation, the promise of extended lifespan, that many have predicted, have not materialized. Although our life expectancy has been increasing–mainly due to an initial drop in child mortality after the Second World War, due to improved public health, water and sewage treatment, and later through the access to vaccinations—life expectancy for those aged 65 years and older has only improved by six years in the last hundred years. In addition, the surge of improved life expectancy received a rude shock in 2014 when statistics showed a reversal. Most countries, especially in some populations in the US and some countries in Europe, were showing a reversal in life expectancy. Whether this is cyclical or a temporary aberration we do not know. But it does signify, without any controversy, that life expectancy is determined by factors that are as fragile as life itself.

Despite the wide debunking of overpopulation theories, leftovers of these theories remain. Especially because of the work of Stanford University Professor Paul Ehrlich—who, together with his wife Anne (although unaccredited)–wrote the best seller 1968 book, *The Population Bomb*—overpopulation remains a strong meme in today's society. Sadly, emerging evidence points in the opposite direction. Humans might be heading towards extinction.

Among humans, both biological capacity (sperm count decline, lower fecundity, obesity rates) and social incentive (high rates of divorce, unemployment, inflexible working conditions, poverty, insecurity, cost of education, health care, housing) are diminishing the desire and ability to reproduce. Within these social changes—populations having fewer children and larger numbers/proportions of older adults—aging is again singled out as the root cause. Since aging does not promote population growth, it is now often seen as a contributing factor to our extinction. Apparently, whether we are heading towards a utopian or a dystopian society, aging again emerges as a reason for dismay.

In our social narrative, in order to save humanity we must now cure aging. Reflecting on the pre-Malthusian arguments that argued for a utopian worldview if we were courageous enough to confront social inequities, we nevertheless fail to address what makes our society uninspiring for young families to bring children into the world. Instead, and similar to the dystopian philosophers of 300 years ago, we are reverting back to science in order to "solve" the problem of aging. Whether aging is necessary for our survival—science has shown that it is—we are now working to ensure that aging is not characterized by frailty and decrepitude.

This social and political context has fed the anti-aging industry. Their solution is simple if somewhat inane: Just do not age. It is no longer enough to interpret aging from an evolutionary biologist's perspective; we must understand the mechanism in order to stop it. In the past, we have looked for the switch in genetics. Some geneticists argue that we have yet to achieve our theoretical lifespan, claiming that we can increase our existing lifespan. Genetic studies have shown that by tweaking one or two genes in non-human animals, lifespan can be increased. But we should not rely too heavily on genetic rescuers.

Genetic determinism.

Genetics have always served as the first line of explanation for physical and sometimes behavioral expressions—as well as for arguments of longevity. The misuse of the term has come to encompass everything that is familial–relating to family influence. But genetic determinism is more specific. It relates to the cause of a physical or biological change determined solely by the presence of a genetic code. The best example of the influence of genes occurs in Mendelian diseases.

Named after the father of genetics, the Austro-German Augustinian friar and abbot Gregor Johann Mendel (1822-1884), Mendelian diseases are determined by a mutation in a single gene causing a disease. Between 1856 and 1863—before genes were discovered in the early

1900s—Mendel was cultivating some 29,000 pea plants. He noticed that peas seem to acquire their characteristics from both parents in a mathematical fashion, with some traits being more dominant than others. Mendel discovered the mathematics of heritability. He found that for every characteristic—a phenotype, an expressed genetic trait—two parts exist, determining how that characteristic is expressed. Now we know that two alleles compose a gene, which determines a physical trait. Mendel's observations indicated that one of these pair as either dominant or recessive. The rest is mathematics; one dominant allele or two recessive alleles to determine a trait. Examples include sickle-cell anemia, Tay-Sachs disease, cystic fibrosis and xeroderma pigmentosa.

Mendelian traits were understood as immutable. If it is caused by a dominant allele then the disease will be expressed. If it is a recessive allele, two alleles are required for the disease to be expressed. Most genetic studies are based on this methodology, but it remains flawed in reasoning. Just because a group had a specific gene and a control group did not, does not define a causal relationship. Just because all "A"s have "B"s does not mean that all "B"s have "A"s.

For more than a century no one tested this foundation of genetics–until now, and the outcome surprised everyone. Up to this study no one looked at the "B"s to see if they have "A"s. In May 2016, in a short eight-page report in Nature Biotechnology, Rong Chen, Stephen Friend and Eric Schadt from the Icahn School of Medicine and their colleagues, overturned a century of dogma about genetic determinism. This small revolution proved to be radical because by association, this also unhinges biological determinism—the belief that biology determines all your traits.

Rong Chen, Stephen Friend and Eric Schadt screened 589,306 people, looking for 874 specific types of genes. They specifically were looking for Mendelian trait genes and identified 584 Mendelian diseases. Thirteen adults were identified as having at least eight severe Mendelian genes. These individuals had either both pairs of a recessive gene, or one of a dominant gene that causes one of eight type of Mendelian disease. But the surprise was that these lucky individuals did not have the diseases. They had the genes but they did not express the diseases. These Mendelian childhood disorders would normally be expected to cause severe disease before the age of 18 years: cystic fibrosis, Smith-Lemli-Opitz syndrome, familial dysautonomia, epidermolysis bullosa simplex, Pfeiffer syndrome, autoimmune polyendocrinopathy syndrome, acampomelic campomelic dysplasia and atelosteogenesis. But for these lucky 13 adults, these genes did not express themselves. They were disease free even though they had the genes for the disease.

This single study has demolished the belief in biological determinism because it argues that all diseases are mediated by something other than genetics.

Amenable diseases

Few diseases are solely determined by genetics. An interaction occurs between the resilience of the body—which decreases with age—and environmental traumas that increase exposure to diseases. A weakened body promotes disease. Genetics seem to control the rate of vulnerability to an ever-present threat of disease and trauma. Comprised resilience as a result of aging is only one side of the equation.

As we discussed earlier with the Gompertz-Makeham equation, two forces act on mortality. One is resilience; the other is the environment (a constant). The environment's importance can be seen in studies that examine how much we can control disease through good public health initiatives.

Joshua Salomon from the Harvard School of Public Health and his colleagues found that although most countries have made substantial progress in reducing mortality over the past two decades, non-fatal disease and injury have not improved to the same degree. Our progress in health outcomes is also slowing in the US, especially with diseases that we can control, and especially for women. Amenable diseases—those that we can prevent and manage—indicate how well health care systems are working. Nearly 20 years ago, the United States was in the middle of other industrialized countries, but countries like Ireland and South Korea improved sharply, leaving the United States lagging even further behind. Across all industrialized countries, because we are living longer, the occurrence of chronic diseases has increased. What we seem to have managed is to push these chronic diseases to emerge later in life. If we truly want to eliminate diseases, how do we go about it? The answer will surprise us.

An international worldwide team of scientists contributed to *The Global Burden of Disease (GBD), Injuries, and Risk Factor study 2013*. The GBD initiative looked at risks for diseases. Some of the risks they looked at explain a large proportion of disease burden. What they found is that basic risks are simple. The top risks include dietary factors, high systolic blood pressure, child and maternal malnutrition, tobacco smoke, air pollution, and obesity. The conclusion is that although variations exist by geography, if we want to help delay half of diseases that kill or disable people then we need to control these risks.   Behavioral, environmental, occupational, and metabolic risks can explain half of global mortality, more than one-third of global disability-adjusted life year (DALY, the number of years lost due to ill health), disability or early death. All these risk factors point to the numerous opportunities for prevention by treating the problem as a public health issue rather than exclusively as a genetic issue.

These risks are reducing our life expectancy and individual life spans. Increasing our life expectancy is logical but not straightforward. Immortalists seek a straightforward solution: finding a cure. It does not matter if our theoretical lifespan is 250 years if our individual lifespan is cut short because of external risks. The immortalists correctly argue that we must eliminate diseases to reach immortality. This is also true on an individual basis. We could all have a true lifespan of hypothetically 250, but it is being cut short because of external risks, e.g. air pollution. Without addressing these risks first, it does not matter what potential we have, or what genetic advances we make; our potential will never be realized.

It seems that the environment moderates all our genes. Effective genes ensure that we survive in the environment we inhabit. In biology, numerous studies look at the translation of the genotype—our genetic makeup—to the phenotype–the final expression of those genes. Many variants in the process can exist. Even if we accept that stunted growth might improve lifespan, other factors might negate such gains. A case in point is a genetically resilient group who are dying early as we saw in Chapter 1 with the Ecuadorian group who suffers from Laron syndrome. Although this group appears to be protected against developing cancer, due to trauma and alcoholism, this Ecuadorian group dies much earlier than other Ecuadorians.

A schism exists between lifespan and theoretical lifespan—that of human behavior.

Why we die

To explain longevity, most of the revolving arguments gravitate toward genetics, but this reliance on an exclusive genetic explanation fails to explain how longevity is achieved. Broader environmental and social issues cannot be ignored or eliminated from the equation. Even in genetic work, the role of the environment is crucial, not just important. This is should not come as a surprise since the sole reason for genes and their modification is to ensure that we adapt to the environment. As a part of this genetic package, longevity is as important as our bigger brain in determining our survival. We die because it allows for the next generation to "have a go" at becoming better adjusted to the environment.

Death does not follow the same rules as a stage play. In most cases, it is a protracted affair. There might be many troughs and peaks, health issues that are survived and healed, or another health issue comes along. This pattern continues for more than a third of one's life. Sometimes the health issue overloads the capacity of the body to cope. But we die because we can no longer resist environmental attacks. The environment takes us out because we become less resistant to it.

Conclusion: Why we are mortal

The development of cooking allowed for easier access to proteins, making it possible for one of the hungriest organs in the body—the brain—to grow. As K-population strategists, a bigger brain improved our ability to learn and store information about our environment. But without a bigger brain needed more nurturing and learning. Longer life expectancy that accompanies a bigger brain allowed us to transfer our critical knowledge from one generation to the next. The survival advantage of a bigger brain required greater longevity. A bigger brain and increased longevity allowed for greater nurturing. This is part of the genetic package. Having a short lifespan negates the advantage of a bigger brain since we cannot transfer knowledge. This combination—longevity and a bigger brain—made humans better at survival. Survival had an effect on younger as well as older age groups. But perhaps we were getting too good at surviving. Perhaps, as some argued, we are prone to overbreeding. Our selfish genes will breed humanity out of existence. And for the first time, mathematicians forayed into this evolving story to clarify the destiny of our population.

The first wave of mathematical theories fueled the fear of over-population. Remnants of the Malthusian revolution are still alive today, despite the lack of evidence for its basic assumptions. The concept of struggle and survival of the fittest defined our headlong selfish desire to reproduce. In this fight and struggle, nature ignores aging because it occurs after the genes have been transmitted–a used tissue, tossed on the course of nature. In this perspective, as we have argued in this chapter, aging became a genetic dustbin, relegated to a mistake of nature. Our hubris, suggesting that reality is at fault, was a first in our civilization. In past centuries, we would have blamed ourselves for annoying the gods. Now we started blaming nature. But the strategy favored by nature is to have fewer children and to nurture them. In order to accomplish this, we needed greater longevity and a bigger brain. If nature could select us for longevity, perhaps we can extend longevity ourselves instead of waiting for nature to determine our fate. In order to understand how our survival package is maintained. We need to appreciate how nature eventually brings about our death. More urgently, can we find the switch that will enable us to turn off death?

———————∞———————

Chapter 3

Search for the Switch

No man is an Island, entire of itself; every man is a piece of the Continent, a part of the main; if a clod be washed away by the sea, Europe is the less, as well as if a promontory were, as well as if a manor of thy friends or of thine own were; any man's death diminishes me, because I am involved in Mankind; And therefore never send to know for whom the bell tolls; It tolls for thee.

–- John Donne, *Meditation XVII, English clergyman & poet (1572 - 1631)*

The search for immortality started with human's first foray into telling stories. Perhaps there was no other story to tell until humans began pondering immortality. The *Epic of Gilgamesh* offers the earliest evidence we have of literature. The earliest writing comes from this collection of clay slabs unearthed in Mosul, Iraq in 1839 by Austen Layard, a British archeologist. These clay slabs contain stories from a much earlier time that tell the story of a King's search for immortality. As we read this poem we become connected by 5,000 years of history. What become known as the *Epic of Gilgamesh* occurred more than 1,800 years before Abraham and the birth of the three main religions in civilization—Judaism, Christianity and Islam. The parallels between the Gilgamesh story and the teachings of Abraham are undisputed—the Garden of Eden, fruit from the tree of knowledge, the Great Flood, a serpent stealing the secret of immortality, redemption, burial and reincarnation, after-life and penitence. Significantly, Abraham's religions have similarly all embraced immortality. Although the Epic warns of "chasing after the wind" (immortality), these religions have, to varying degrees, accepted our immortal status through the creation of a soul. A very close parallel exists between the concept of the soul and the concept of immortality. The development of the soul mirrors the transformative change in how we see our gods.

From Greek and Roman times, when gods were seen as aloof and distant, to the god of Abraham that is personal and intimate, we can chart how humans made gods to behave more like themselves. We accomplished this humanity by creating a soul, a remnant of god that exists within us. It is impossible to get more human than a god that shares your humanity. The soul is the test of our moral worth. Stephen Cave, in his excellent book on *Immortality*, makes an enlightened and provocative case for the soul helping to "sell" immortality to humans. He argues that the soul was part of a much more radical change in human thought. The relationship that we have with gods has changed to reflect our own individualistic and narcissistic development in modern society. From the gods of ancient Mesopotamia and Egypt—one of the earliest civilizations in world history, which began 3500BC—3100BC, followed by the religions of India and China (2700BC-1900BC), and the ancient Greeks and Romans (1000BC). The gods before Abraham were distant, disengaged and unfeeling.

From these religions, three folklores evolved that have dictated our quest for immortality. These folklore stories have guided our search for immortality, and have tainted our view of our survival package. We have forgotten that death is part of the nature of life. But because we started to believe that immortality is assured after death, all we can think about now is to find the death switch in order to turn it off. We can have immortality here on earth and we had stories and folklore to promote this ambition of ours.. These folklores relate to a time when people lived longer (Antediluvian), lived longer in other parts of the world (Hyperborean), and where we can apply a compound that makes us younger (Fountain of Youth).

Three Themes in Folklore

Folklore—cultural beliefs—and science play a duet in this field, feeding off of each other. Some folklore have promoted some scientific beliefs, while in contrast some scientific discoveries rejuvenate long held cultural beliefs. Mirko Dražen Grmek, wrote a book–one of the hidden gems of gerontology covering a period from 384 BC to 1957 Grmek's forgotten monograph provides a clear linear history of gerontology that focuses primarily on geriatrics but also has great insight into social and physical aspects of getting older (homes, hospital and asylums.) Together with Gerald

Gruman, who focused exclusively on the prolongation of life—living longer—these two early monographs provide a succinct historical perspective of how ancient beliefs continue to influence our scientific thinking today.

Antediluvian

The Antediluvian folklore—referring to a time before the ancient floods—has seen many interpretations, across all religions, continents, languages and cultures (including Hollywood). Flood stories emanate from around the world and throughout history. Mark Isaak documents a few hundred stories where floods are mentioned. All great pre-historical texts, including the first known human literature, the Sumerian saga of Gilgamesh, refers to how the god Enlil warned the priest-king Ziusudra "Long of Life" of the coming flood. Ziusudra was instructed to build a great ship to save his family and other animals. Although now ascribed to the Bible, this theme runs through varied cultures, geographies and time periods. The story of the flood remains one of the most common features of religions throughout the world.

Longevity folklore is best described in the Book of Genesis (5:27) when Methuselah was said to have lived 969 years, dying in the year of the Great Flood. It is here that the myth emerged that the flood was a turning point and that humankind lost its ability to live much longer. Although Methuselah's age is an error in translating units of time—taking one month as a year—the name Methuselah remains the catchphrase for longevity. An error in translating age and a moral story of punishment without redemption created the Antediluvian myth. A myth that we lived longer in the past, but lost such an ability as punishment for our wickedness. Today, the story of long-lived humans before the flood—

aside from some religious sects—is scientifically recognized for what it is, a parable and a myth.

Hyperborean

Referring to the belief that people live longer in some parts of the world—ostensibly at the edge of the world where the boreal lights light up the sky. These boreal lights are known as 'Aurora borealis' in the north and 'Aurora Australis' in the south. A classic example of Hyperborean belief appeared in the 1973 issue of National Geographic, when Alexander Leaf gave a detailed account of his journeys to regions of purported long-living people: Hunzas in Pakistan, Abkhazians in the Soviet Union, and Ecuadorians in Vilcabamba. According to this article, despite poor sanitation, prevalence of infectious diseases, high infant mortality, illiteracy, and a lack of modern public health and medical care, there were ten times more centenarians in these countries than in most Western countries.

It did not help that the first ever paperback, published in 1933, was the novel *Lost Horizon* by English writer James Hilton. It tells the story of a group of travelers whose small plane crash landed somewhere in the Himalayas and they were saved by an order of monks who seemed to be immortal. This book was the origin of Shangri-La, a fictional utopian lamasery high in the mountains of Tibet, which was believed to be the home of immortals. But as much as this was fiction, so was Alexander Leaf's story in the National Geographic.

Leaf eventually admitted his mistake. He went back to verify the story and in the process exposed the lies that engendered it. The locals told Leaf that they wanted to make him happy and give him what he wanted. His mistake was in accepting their self-reported ages, given in order to please him, as fact. The Hyperborean folklore died a slow death with the advent of easy and cheap flights to distant countries. In the 1950s and 60s, such Hyperborean stories slowly disappeared. But the wish to believe in a perfect place where we live a long and fruitful life remains strong. As recently as 2009, Scientific American published a remarkable age claim by Sakhan Dosova of Kazakhstan who was said to be 130 years when she died. Further investigation identified a lack of early-life documentation and subsequent evidence of falsification.

This fascination with very older adults is not new. As early as the 1700s, researchers were becoming interested in centenarians—people that live up to and beyond 100 years of age. Then in the 1930's, the US Bureau of the Census compared the proportion of centenarians in different countries. Despite the historically unreliability of longevity claims, claims of clusters of centenarians persisted. One of the first of such studies was conducted because it was atypical, a cluster exhibiting extreme male longevity in Sardinia. After corroborating the findings using rigid methodology, this finding of a cluster of centenarians led to the identification of other such clusters. The Hyperborean story would have been dead and buried if not for Dan Buettner, who as the lead explorer. Buettner rejuvenated the theme in a 2009 National Geographic article where he referred to communities that have a high concentration of centenarians as "Blue Zones." The term Blue Zones comes from the blue pen used by the demographer on the project, Michel Poulain, to mark the cluster of centenarians on a map of Sardinia, which was the first place that they looked at.

To date, five "Blue Zone" communities throughout the world have been identified. These are Sardinia, Italy;; Okinawa, Japan; Loma Linda, California; Costa Rica's isolated Nicoya Peninsula; and Ikaria, a Greek island. Other such small clusters remain to be uncovered throughout the world.

With this discovery, the Hyperborean folklore became more specific and contained. These clusters of centenarians are fairly small, consisting of some 20 individuals. Although centenarians are found across the globe, distinct clusters of centenarians only exist in traditional communities—an indication that geography plays an important role in reaching extreme old age. We do not find this cohort grouped among the very rich, among the highly educated, or among one specific ethnic group, or only among women—we find them only in specific geographic clusters. Although they share certain types of activities, attitudes and diet, not everyone who shares these characteristics lives to extreme ages. If aging occurs as a random event, unaffected by external variables, clusters of older adults should be equitable across geography and strata of individuals, based purely upon population density. But we do not see that. Instead, we find distinct geographic clusters only. We do not find such clusters only in rich countries, specific ethnic groups, educational and income strata, or gender. We find these blue zones only in distinct geographies.

Fountain of Youth

And last, but certainly not least, the most tenacious and pervasive folklore, that of the "Fountain of Youth." This story refers to the ability to rejuvenate, and regress to an earlier younger self by ingesting or administering a substance. The fountain of youth encapsulates all of those psychological tricks used to lull us–that everything can be corrected and we can reclaim our youth. It has become the magic bullet, a panacea, and a cure-all. Although incorrectly associated with Ponce De Leon a 1500s Spanish explorer in

Florida, the concept of rejuvenating balm has a much longer history, going back, again to the story of Gilgamesh. Gilgamesh was looking for the plant of immortality, and although he found it, he lost again to a snake—who now sheds his skin and rejuvenates itself. Subsequent stories follow a similar pattern. In the 300s BC Alexander the Great describes a "river of paradise." A river that washes away old age to reveal a younger wet self. But the true search for immortality was never as zealotry conducted as the first emperor of China.

Ying Zheng militarily and administratively consolidated all of China in 221 BC. Because of this great power, he failed to accept that he was mortal like other human beings.. He did everything in his control to stay alive and gain immortality. His fixation—helped by ingesting mercury—eventually killed him at age 49. Just before he died, however, he sent his priest Xu Fu to look for the elixir of life.

The story goes that after equipping Xu Fu with 60 ships and around 5,000 crew—including 3,000 virgin boys and girls—Xu Fu set out on his search for the mystical Penglai Mountain (most likely Mount Fuji in Japan). At the second attempt, Xu Fu never returned. Legend claims that Xu Fu and his entourage reached Japan, colonized it and, the legend goes, transformed Japan by introducing new farming techniques along with iron and bronze implements. The early death of the first emperor of China did not deter the proliferation of stories of the fountain of youth.

Europeans in the Middle Ages believed in the mythical king Prester John, whose kingdom contained a fountain of youth and a river of gold. In the 1300s Roger Bacon brought two of these folklores together by arguing that the Methuselah prowess of living up to 900-years would be restored through alchemy.

Francis Bacon, the father of the scientific method in the early 1600s in an issue of *The New Atlantis* published after his death, argued for organ replacement and the "Water of Paradise." He wrote *The Cure of Old Age and Preservation of Youth* that promoted "the prolongation of life, the restitution of youth to some degree, the retardation of age."

The Fountain of Youth theme persists today, embraced and promoted by the Anti-Aging movement. As elusive as the fountain of youth has been, it is our desire for youth that still nourishes this particular fountain of myth—propagated by ignorance and a series of misunderstandings about aging. One of the arguments made by the anti-aging movement is that no lifespan exists, no limit to how many years we can live. To make such an argument they use the increase in life expectancy as proof that we are inexorably moving towards pushing the barrier of death to older and older ages. But we are not. The misuse of statistics clouds the discussion.

The first misunderstanding involves the difference between lifespan and life expectancy. While lifespan is the maximum number of years humans have ever reached, life expectancy is the age at which half of a population is expected to die. No single study exists that validates the extension of lifespan in humans. Not one. The much-touted increase in life expectancy is due nearly exclusively to reduced child mortality and virtually little to do with advances in treatment of older adults. In fact, if half of a population survives to 200 years of age, the life expectancy will nevertheless remain the same. Life expectancy is not determined by how long people live, but how young they die since it records the age of death when the middle of a group dies.

In the last century, life expectancy of 65 has increased by only 5.7 years in the United States. This indicates that public health and medicine exert little influence on life expectancy, other than promoting child health. And child health is important, of and by itself, because it increases the number of children who reach older ages–which dramatically increases life expectancy.

Despite the lack of evidence of the prolongation of human life, themes that promote elixirs to reverse aging pervade commonly-held beliefs. Bad science, from both sides of the spectrum—resulted in scientific establishments and peripheral fringe organizations and individuals who promote this delusion. Studies showing improved life expectancy for a group that follows a specific diet are rife with methodological faults. Despite these shortfalls, such evidence is sometimes elevated as new elixirs of longevity. By looking at one specific diet change rather than multiple aspects of life, what we get is unconnected associations. Humans' complex biology achieves a sophisticated homeostasis and balance that vary tremendously as we age. Single factors are unlikely to affect functioning. Numerous studies do, however, show improvement through the use of single supplements. Through faulty methodology combined with over-generalization, these studies build a false edifice of longevity elixirs. Welcome to the world of anti-aging..

Immortality Business

In 2004, the co-founders of the Chicago-based American Academy of Anti-Aging Medicine (A4M) sued two academic professors for confirming a truth upon which scientists around the world agree, that you cannot reverse aging. These were not just two ordinary professors. The suit named S. Jay Olshansky, a sociologist and professor in the School of Public Health at the University of Illinois at

Chicago; and Thomas Perls, a physician and professor of medicine at Boston University School of Medicine. Olshansky, has published more than 109 papers in refereed journals, 33 books and book chapters, and numerous other presentations and publications, while Perls has published more than 100 papers in refereed journals, 14 textbook chapters and two books. These established academicians reported how simplistic the anti-aging message is—and that it is wrong. The story escalated when Olshansky awarded A4M the "silver fleece"—a designation meant to shame medical professionals who claim they have invented ways of reversing aging. The suit also alleges that at a 2004 A4M conference, Olshansky left a bottle of vegetable oil labeled "snake oil" for Ronald M. Goldman and Ronald M. Klatz, as the joint owners of A4M.

The suit for $240 million alleged that the professors—by criticizing anti-aging practices–a topic for which they are renowned and have published extensively on—undermined A4M's scientific credibility, "and by so doing harms the business prospects of the founders." On Nov. 17 2005, this suit ended in a settlement, with neither side paying damages nor the other's costs. If the University of Chicago had not supported these two professors in the suit, such threats would bankrupt most academicians.

Among many of the criticisms, the authors argued that an estimated third of all growth hormone prescriptions in the U.S. are written for non-FDA-approved uses. Growth hormone might make you feel and look young, but it is not to be confused with reversing the aging process. Feeling and looking good is not the same as being younger, but then we have been deceived on this point for far too long. Welcome to the world of false hopes and the peddlers of immortality.

Gurus of Immortality

Aging is a great business. The American Academy of Anti-Aging Medicine (A4M) cloaks the area with a scientific mantle. Although they base their assertions on scientifically robust individual studies, in most cases, these studies become willfully unreliable and invalid when generalized to humans. When such deception fails, it seems that they then rely on lawyers to silence dissent. The path of deception is littered with such gurus of immortality, with a singular outcome: failure. The following is a list of people who promised exceptional long life, health and vitality. In most cases the health issue at which they directed their magic was what killed them. The most common age of death for these aspiring immortalists is around 75-80 years of age. Although this is a reasonable old age this is by no means exceptional. Any professional group of people will have a similar life expectancy. The litany of names that fail to attain immortality is frequently updated:

- Adelle Davis (1904-1974), who often said she never saw anyone get cancer who drank a quart of milk a day, as she did—died of bone cancer at age 70.

- Paavo Airola (1918-1983) promoted natural healing through a diet of nutritious, whole foods and holistic medicine. He died of a stroke at the age of 64.

- Jim Fixx (1932-1984), who championed the health benefits of running and claimed that regular running offered virtual immunity to heart disease, died of a heart attack while jogging at age 52.

- Nathan Pritikin (1915-1985), after being diagnosed with heart disease, advocated regular exercise and a low fat, high-fiber diet. He committed suicide at age 69 while suffering from leukemia.

- T.C. Fry (1926-1996) was a leader of the Natural Hygiene movement in the US who died at the age of 70, of a pulmonary embolism.

- Robert Atkins (1930-2003), the proponent of a high protein, low carbohydrate diet, died of a brain injury.

- Roy Walford (1924-2004) a proponent of caloric restriction as a means to extending life, died of Lou Gehrig's disease at age 79.

- Robert E. Kowalski (1942-2007) a cholesterol guru who wrote *8 Steps to a Healthy Heart* (Grand Central Publishing, 1994) died at the age of 65 from a pulmonary embolism.

- Alan Mintz (1938-2007) a controversial proponent of using human growth hormone—an anabolic steroid—died at age 69 from complications of a brain biopsy. Brain cancer seems to be a particular risk to anabolic steroid use.

- Michel Montignac (1944-2010) focused on the glycemic index and the distinction between good and bad carbohydrates. Montignac died of prostate cancer at the age of 66.

- Stuart Berger (1954-1994), who advocated vitamins, minerals and exercise, died of a heart attack at 40. His corpse weighed 365lbs. five years before his death he wrote *"Forever Young — 20 Years Younger in 20 Weeks: Dr. Berger's Step-by-Step Rejuvenation Program,"* (William Morrow & Company, 1989)

- Michio Kushi (1926-2014) advocated a macrobiotic diet and wrote *The Cancer Prevention Diet.* He died of colon cancer at 88, while his wife died of cervical cancer at 78.

- Wilfred (1907-1982) and Evan Shute (1905-1978)– Canadian cardiologist brothers, promoted the use of Vitamin E to combat heart disease. In 1981, while continuing to lecture on the prevention of heart disease with Vitamin E, Wilfred developed heart disease. He died after a bypass operation at the age of 75. Evan preceded him at age 73.

- Jerome Irving Rodale (1898-1971), founder of *Prevention* magazine emphasized prevention of disease while advocating for an organic diet. He died at age 72 of a heart attack on camera while being interviewed by Dick Cavett for a taped TV episode

- George Ohsawa (1893-1966), inventor of Macrobiotics ("the way of long life") had a more comprehensive approach–embodying spiritual as well as nutritional values. He died of lung cancer at 73.

- Vilhjalmur Stefansson (1879-1962) a Canadian ethnologist spent more than a decade with the Inuit and ate almost exclusively fish and seal meat (often raw or fermented), and almost no vegetables. He later developed cardiovascular disease, dying of a stroke at the age of 82.

Other entrepreneurs that made a living selling their technique for healthy living–had a more realistic aim. They aspired to live life to the full, doing what they loved doing, being healthy and active, eating good quality produce and being active.

- Paul Bragg (1895-1976) an American nutritionist, promoted deep breathing, water fasts, organic foods, drinking distilled water, juicing, exercise, listening to one's body, and many other techniques as methods of prolonging life span. He died at the age of 81, apparently from a heart attack.

- Norman Walker (1886-1985), a British businessman, advocated juicing and drinking fresh raw vegetable and fruits–both to regain and to maintain one's health. He died at the age of 99.

- Jack Lalanne (1914-2011), an American fitness and diet guru, promoted exercise for older adults and those with disabilities as a way of maintaining active. He died at the age of 96 from pneumonia.

Some nutritional experts often assume that living a healthy life extends lifespan. Eat well and you can live forever, or at least up to 120 years. It seems that wherever you turn there is a new fad for eating "right" and a new savior to tell us how to do it. In reality, older adults exhibit unique dietary deficiencies. Especially in the United States we see two polarizing realities. On the one hand, we have an obesity epidemic. More than one-third of older adults aged 65 and over were obese in 2007–2010, a percentage that is increasing, especially for men. Minority older women tend to show greater obesity, while minority older men tend to be less obese than Whites.

In contrast to this growing obesity epidemic among older adults, a different group of seniors are becoming increasing under-nourished. More than one in five of older adults experience food insecurity—not know where their next meal is coming from. Within this group a small percentage—about one in 20 people—experience hunger in a given year. Some older adults go hungry due to poverty, while others eat inappropriately. The constant scolding by self-identified experts to eat well, while bombarding us with ever-changing advice, confuses even the most informed of consumers. But science shows that apart from reducing the risk of ill health, good nutrition is–like air–necessary but not proportional in its positive effect on aging.

Such self-proclaimed experts, holders of immorality truths and those who claim to hold the nutritional secret to long life, share one common characteristic—they are all dead. The real truth is that scientists know very little about diet in older age. The oldest person that has ever lived, Jeanne Louise Calment, might have some secrets herself. When she died in 1977, Calment was 122 years and 164 days. She started smoking when she was 21 years old and did not stop until the age of 117. She ate nearly two pounds of chocolate every week, and drank port wine. She ascribed her longevity to olive oil, which she said she poured all her food and rubbed onto her skin. Despite the luxury of such daily habits, it is likely that marrying into money had a significant influence on her longevity. Circumstances made it possible for her to never having to work and to instead she lived a leisured life, pursuing hobbies like tennis, cycling, swimming, roller skating, piano and opera. Being economically secure allows you to survive to old age, but we still do not know what promotes extreme long life. The search for the elusive switch continues. Which might be strange conclusion to admit since we only have to look at the local grocery store to find the answer: Supplements.

Supplements

Pick up the paper or open any news item in your browser and you are likely to be assaulted with the latest supplement that has been proven to promote longevity, delay dementia, or make you younger. Such is our longing for the fountain of youth.

Most of these individual supplements have very interesting histories. Their relationship with longevity is tenuous at best, but nevertheless not totally without merit. Just because we do not understand whether, or how they work, does not diminish the fervor with which some supplements are promoted. The problem with establishing the validity of these supplements—whether they work— relates to the method of study. The scientific method of identifying causality is not as straightforward as the public assumes. Many factors should be considered (and eliminated from confusing the results), especially when looking at longevity. Examples of this type of thinking exist in the study of longevity. As with earlier studies, involving testosterone—which eventually resulted in the birth of the field of endocrinology—these new outcomes are not yet understood. If history has any bearing on our investigation, it is primarily because we are listening to individual tones and not appreciating the overall composition of the music. Staying with the example of testosterone, we need to understand the mechanism in order to appreciate the role these supplements play in extending longevity…or not.

To make sense of the enormous field of longevity supplements, we might identify these underlying processes and come to a more fruitful understanding of the quest for immortality. The development of a diagram to summarize these results might expose an underlying pattern.

Diagram 1 identifies some of the most important supplements in use today to increase longevity. Supplements aid longevity through specific mechanisms. The basic mechanisms are whether they involve tumor suppression or sleep enhancement. Other "effects mechanisms" are more technical, as with protein production or promoting mitochondria function. Evidence exists that these supplements promote each of these mechanisms. Independently these mechanisms can be useful at promoting longevity by preventing early death. Whatever the mediating mechanism, the ultimate overarching mechanisms can be summarized under Caloric Restriction and Anti-Oxidants. These two mechanisms are offered as the main reasons why these supplements work.

Diagram 1: A Selection of Individual Supplements (on the far right and far left) and Possible Mechanisms for Improved Longevity in the shaded circles.

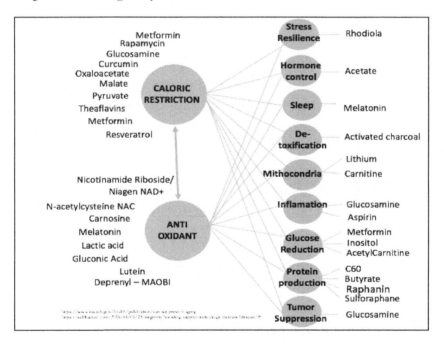

This is neither a comprehensive nor systematic review of supplements. It reflects the most popular supplements—there are many more—and categorizes them by their potential effectiveness. The significance of this analysis is that all of these supplements seem, at some point, to promote two main mechanisms for promoting longevity, that of caloric restriction and/or use of an anti-oxidant. And these two ways that these supplements likely work are related to each other. There is a connection between caloric restriction and anti-oxidants. It appears that caloric restriction might prolong life by reducing free radicals.

If we look at how caloric restriction works in increasing longevity, we find that a surprising feedback system is in place. A feedback system instructing the body to become more efficient. We also find that some of the genetic variance in longevity also parallels the effects of caloric restriction.

Caloric Restriction

Caloric Restriction (CR) refers to an overall 20 to 40 percent reduction of total caloric intake. Calories are ways of evaluating the energy stored in food on the basis of how much energy the item of food has. One calorie is approximate amount of energy needed to raise the temperature of one gram of water by one degree Celsius at a pressure of one atmosphere. CR works not only as a reduction in the overall intake of calories, but seems to work by engaging the body in other surprising ways. These other ways are mostly unknown.

Recently the definition of CR has included a broader scope of interventions, including short-term starvation (2-3 days of not eating, but drinking water), periodic fasting (one or two days a week/month of not eating solids), fasting-mimetic diets (reducing individual's caloric intake down to 34 to 54 percent of normal, with a specific composition of proteins, carbohydrates, fats and micronutrients), intermittent fasting (one day of not eating solids, or just eating one meal a day), normo-caloric diets with planned deficiencies (which are normal diets modified by restricting particular macronutrients–substances required in relatively large amounts by living organisms: proteins, carbohydrates, etc. examples include methionine-, and tryptophan-restricted diets), and time-restricted feeding (only eating at certain times of the day, for example five hours before going to sleep and having at least 12 hours between dinner and breakfast). Most of these techniques have shown some positive outcome. This outcome is unexpected if we are looking only at calories, since some of these diet actually increase calorie intake. So the underlying mechanism of why these methods work is leading us away from purely caloric intake to possibly a shock mechanism. Caloric Restriction acts as a shock to the system and initiates a series of changes that are beneficial for longevity.

Clive McCay initially discovered CR in 1935 in mice. More than 80 years of research has resulted, showing that CR increases the lifespan in yeast, insects, and in non-human primates.   In humans, CR is still undergoing testing, although initial results suggest that prevention of age-related diseases may eventually result in the prolongation of life. The mechanism seems to emulate the genetic work of life prolongation, in that the CR elicits a hormesis event—a low level stressor that stimulates positive response. Similar to the adage "once bitten twice shy," hormesis involves the response from the body to low-level stress that activates a positive counter response. Hormesis has long been shown to have a positive affect on lifespan. At the turn of the century, Wheeler Davey with General Electric Company reported that low doses of ionizing radiation increased the lifespan of the Confused Beetle. Later John Cork confirmed this study in 1957.

More recently in a 2015 randomized study—CALERIE: Comprehensive Assessment of the Long-term Effects of Reducing Intake of Energy—involving 250 healthy adults, reported that a two-year quarter reduction in caloric intake provides health benefits, such as reduced inflammation and reduced chance of getting diabetes, heart disease or stroke. According to Edward Masoro with the University of Texas, this could only be brought about by three mechanisms that determine how CR works. Similar to diagram 1, he includes decrease in free radicals (oxidative stress), control of sugar and insulin in the blood, and finally hormesis (which we will discuss in the next chapter.)

Oxidative stress refers to the creation of radicals in the body. Radicals are molecules with missing electrons making them unbalanced and they go around the body looking to replace the lost electron. All radicals are free, meaning they are scavengers and circulating around the body, attempting to attach to another electron. Since electrons prefer to be in pairs, radicals try to steal electrons from another atom. This is what makes them "free." Stealing electrons, however, results in a dangerous chain reaction of "tag–you're it."

Molecules lose an electron as byproduct of body functions (metabolism), when the body changes oxygen and proteins into energy. The more you use your body, such as exercise, the higher the number of radicals that you create. The primary contender for an explanation of aging is the accumulation of these toxic by-products. Although exercise creates more radicals, exercise also makes your body more efficient at dealing with radicals. It is a balance—too much or too little activity is dangerous. Radicals when generated in excess become highly toxic.

Anti-Oxidants

Once released, these free radicals physically puncture and destroy neighboring cells. All activity in the body releases free radicals. Antioxidants trap these free radicals by giving them an electron to attach to and therefore diffuse them. This raised hopes that we could prevent slow damage from radicals simply by adding antioxidants to the diet. However, so far, studies do not support this expectation.

Sometimes radicals can also be caused by external factors, such as pollutants, tobacco, smoke, drugs, foreign substances, or radiation. When a person's antioxidant defense mechanism cannot cope with the volume of radicals, it causes oxidative stress. Radicals react chemically with fat, protein, and DNA around them. This is not good—since then radicals can start acting like the proverbial bull in a china shop. Radicals can damage essential cells in the body.

Many types of radicals exist. The most common form of free radicals is known as reactive oxygen species (ROS), referring to the chemically reactive chemical species containing oxygen. Oxygen has two unpaired electrons, and in processing oxygen the mitochondria (the energy generator in the cell) produces ROS. This is a normal by-product of cell activity. The name oxygen derives from the Greek oxys-, "acid," and -genes, "producer". So, despite oxygen being one of the most essential chemicals for life on Earth, it has been known to be somewhat toxic.

It is perplexing that in most cases, ROS protect humans from microbes. ROS surrounds bacteria or viruses and starves them to death. The problem emerges when the body is under stress, producing too much ROS, which then becomes toxic. These by-products include peroxides, superoxide, hydroxyl radical, and singlet oxygen. In response the body uses many enzymes, vitamins and other small molecules as antioxidants and by combining with the radical, transforming themselves into less toxic substances.

The problem with radicals is that at lower doses, they are useful to the body. Sometimes even at high doses ROS has tumor-suppressing attributes. Again, it seems that the body operates a finely tuned balancing act. Depending on the concentration and conditions, radicals might result in beneficial or harmful effects, depending on our body's metabolic condition. Such a nuanced interpretation of the effect of radicals on the body, deflect from the good vs. bad judgment that we seek. We continue looking for binary answers.

The enduring ease with which we accept the fountain of youth narrative can be measured by the growth of the supplement industry worldwide. According to a 2017 report by Grand View research, the global dietary supplement market is expected to reach $278 million by 2024. A quarter of this will be in the United States. The main players are some heavy hitters of the pharmacology industry: Amway Corporation, Pfizer Pharmaceuticals, Abbott Laboratories, Herbalife International, ADM, DuPont, and Carlyle Group.

The search for the biological mechanisms of aging–the switch that will eventually turn death off–has been elusive so far, although not for a lack of trying. The U.S. National Institute on Aging has three areas of focus: genetics, metabolism (including anti-oxidants and hormesis), and the immune system (mainly examining stress). Although many promises have been made, few of these hypotheses adequately explain aging. Perhaps aging is more complex that we want to admit. If this is the case, then the search for switches should be seen as a prelude to a more comprehensive understanding of aging.

Telomere Theory

In the late 1800s, the German biologist August Weismann correctly guessed the existence of a cell-division limit that later developed into the Telomeric Theory (as developed by Leonard Hayflick and others). Weismann later addressed the differences between germ cells (eggs and sperm) and the somatic cells (all other types of cells), writing about "…the perishable and vulnerable nature of the soma." This concept directly contributed to Thomas Kirkwood's Disposable Soma Theory.   The two theories—Telomeric and Disposable Soma—although independent—provide some of the most hopeful approaches to date that explain biological aging. The idea has been, and remains, that if we can understand the biological mechanism, perhaps a switch that we can tweak will adjust or even eliminate aging.

Our mortality is a modern concept. At the turn of the century we still clung to the belief that some people were immortal—or very long lived—and living in some remote place of the world. We also clung to the belief that our cells are immortal and that we behave in ways that kill these cells. All these beliefs imply that we are immortal except that we are doing something wrong. We remained stained with the original sin that brought us mortality.

In the 1900s, the reign of the French surgeon Alexis Carrel—a 1912 Nobel Prize winner in surgery—grew chicken cells in petri dishes for a number of decades. He believed, as did the rest of the world, that cells are immortal. We do bad things to them to kill them. In folklore, such sin is pervasive. It was assumed that humans did something wrong to deserve death—such as eating from the forbidden tree; or the Taoist's loss of Ching; or Aristotle's loss of innate moisture. Our belief system held that under the right circumstances, our cells do not die, and therefore we will not die.

Alexis Carrel's hold on science was absolute. The infamous French surgeon had developed methods for connecting blood vessels and conducted successful kidney transplants on dogs. Carrel was a pioneer of organ transplantation. Working with Charles Lindbergh, he is even credited with developing an early version of an artificial heart. Later in life, while at the Rockefeller Institute for Medical Research in New York, there was a sense of mysticism within his laboratories. All laboratory staff wore ninja-looking black lab scrubs, covering their head all the way down to their feet. With black gloves the only human exposure was through slits for their eyes.   No reason required this attire, other than a sense of control that Carrel exerted over his staff. Peering through small slits for their eyes, these lab technicians kept the chicken heart cells alive in petri dishes for more than 20 years. Even though it was impossible to replicate his cell culture's immortality, laboratories throughout the world endorsed the belief that cells are immortal. Until Leonard Hayflick's observations caused science to question this belief.

In 1961, going against scientific thinking at the time, biologist Leonard Hayflick and virologist Paul Moorhead noticed that their cell cultures were dying after replicating a certain number of times. Hayflick demonstrated that normal human fibroblast cells divide about 70 times in 3 percent oxygen—the same as human internal conditions—before discontinuing to replicate. Cells die. The limit to cells being able to replicate has become known as the Hayflick Limit. Refuting the idea that normal cells are immortal and establishing a biological basis for lifespan. This Hayflick Limit has earned the crown as the primary theory explaining human lifespan, and for the first time it was suggested that we might be engineered to die.

Despite an ever-increasing life expectancy, where people are living longer, an invisible wall still exists, one that we cannot live beyond—this is the lifespan. No one has broken through the ceiling established by the longest living person, Jean Louis Calment at 122 years. The best explanation we have of an absolute and static lifespan is the concept of the Hayflick Limit—a genetic program that stops cells from replicating. It is a beautiful concept, that every cell in our body is engineered to die.

The mechanism for the "Hayflick Limit" was not yet known at the time Hayflick made his observation. But a Russian scientist Alexey Olovnikov hypothesized in 1971 how such a process might work. While waiting for a train at a terminal, Olovnikov noticed that the engine of the train does not go right to the edge of the track. The end of the track remains untouched by the engine's wheels. In a moment of inspiration, he thought of how genetic material is copied—the process where our DNA is translated into a copy of itself—and understood that the enzyme that does the copying, must miss the end of the DNA when it copies it. He called these genes at the end of the DNA, 'telogenes'. With each cell division one of these telogenes would be sacrificed until all 50 are used up and the DNA unravels. These end bits hold the genetic material together, and much like an aglet on a shoelace, once the little plastic wrap erodes, then the rest of the shoe lace starts to fray. Writing in the 1973 issue of the Journal of Theoretical Biology, Olovnikov understood the implication of this biological ticking time bomb that causes "various disorders of age of the ageing of multicellular organisms." Calling it the theory of 'marginotomy,' he also assumed that cancer cells are governed by the same mechanism and that there should be a substance that protects the telogenes. He was right on both counts.

This protective substance has been identified as an enzyme called 'telomerase.' In addition, Olovnikov correctly predicted the circular form of bacteria's genome as a means of protecting its DNA from shortening. Olovnikov's elegant theory remained hidden in obscurity. But it was not until much later in 1984 that Elizabeth Blackburn and Carol Greider—winning the 2009 Nobel Prize in Biology—confirmed this process. They found evidence for telogenes—which they identified as proteins and re-named telomeres—at the end of the DNA that get shorter with every division until they get too short to allow for further replication. This telomeric theory identifies the mechanism for the Hayflick Limit. A ticking time bomb that Hayflick identified and which Olovnikov theorized and which Blackburn and Greider validated. Each cell has an expiration date that is determined by the number of times it can replicate itself. Once that counter reaches zero, the cell dies.

In general, telomeres are prone to shrink every time the cell divides. Aging is the main factor for telomere shortening. Telomeres also react to stress, an unhealthy diet, excessive intake of alcohol, smoking, lack of exercise and other behaviors we associate as health risks, including caregiving stress. Shortened telomeres are related to an increased risk of cancer, heart disease and a series of other diseases. Here was a mechanism that not only explains aging, but can also hold the answer to stopping it. As eloquent as this theory is however, large variances exist in correlating telomere length with aging and with lifespan.

First, telomeres are not proportional to longevity. Three main arguments have evolved that dispel the notion that telomeres explain lifespan. Working in comparative biology, Nuno Gomez from the University of Texas Southwestern Medical Center and his colleagues undertook the largest comparative study involving more than 60 mammalian species. They reported that telomere length inversely correlates with lifespan, while telomerase (an enzyme that promotes the growth of telomeres) correlates with the physical size of the body of the species.

The second argument comes from Leonard Hayflick himself, who–writing in his 1994 book *How and Why We Age*—speculated that assuming human fibroblasts endure 70 divisions, more than enough divisions for several lifetimes. Biologically it is feasible that individual cells in our body can maintain their level of division and renewal for at least 150 years. And still, no one has lived beyond 122 years. But the dislike for the telomeric theory comes from the supplement-peddling industry itself. Since each cell has its own switch, with over 37 trillion cells in our body, there are a lot of switches to control. This does not bode well for a binary answer or a quick supplement infusion to stop these clocks ticking.

In 2016, Teresa Rivera and her colleagues with the Salk Institute reported that it is not just short telomeres that cause problems, but also long telomeres. Having long telomeres created instability in the cells and in most cases caused cancer. This was termed as the "Goldilocks Effect"– not too small, not too big, but just right. It seems that telomeres do not provide us with a complete picture. Although the Hayflick Limit predicts that there must be a lifespan—an upper limit to longevity—evidence suggests that that limit has yet to be achieved. This has opened the door to search for another biological mechanism, the ever-elusive switch that controls longevity. One way around this conundrum—that we cannot control all of the telomeres in our body—is to replace aging cells with new ones. The body already has such a system in place, called stem cells.

The third argument against the telomeric theory of lifespan comes from the Italian biologist Giuseppina Tesco and her colleagues in 1998—refuting earlier studies—found that fibroblast taken from centenarians showed no difference in the number of replications compared to cells from younger donors. This finding can however be explained by another intervening process which retains the integrity of the telomere. It could be that within the body, cells can be replaced with new ones—rather than simply renewed. Adult stem cells have been identified in many organs and tissues of older adults, including brain, bone marrow, peripheral blood, teeth, heart, gut, liver, blood vessels, skeletal muscle, skin, ovarian epithelium, and testis. They are thought to reside in a "stem cell niche" which is a specific area within each tissue. We all have these and yet some of us seem to use them up more rapidly. Perhaps we started with fewer stem cells, or the environment that we live in degraded them faster. Older adults are more likely to have used up their supply of stem cell or experienced more stressors that damaged their stem cells. Once stem cells run out or become damaged, the body cannot replace them. But a limit also exists for the utility of our endowed stem cells. In the meantime they can replace certain fibroblasts in older people, making them seem young.

Stem Cells

Stem cells are undifferentiated cells called "multipotent cells." They are like the joker in a pack of cards, and in our body they can be transformed to any type of cell that we need. Although they still renew themselves through replication (mitosis), they remain undefined until they are ready to be used by the body. Stem cell theory of aging would argue that either the stem cells have been degraded through age or exposure to toxins (oxidative stress, radiation, or other assault), or they are simply used-up and their supply depleted.

The argument for the importance of stem cells in aging comes from dementia research. The first sign of dementia is the loss of olfactory senses. The sense of smell is accomplished through our olfactory system–an old system in our biological development. This olfactory system has a direct path to the brain. With humans, the system starts with the nose and ends a short distance away at the base of our brain. Olfactory receptors, with very thin fibers, run from the roof of the nasal cavity through perforations in the skull ending in the olfactory bulbs, which are a pair of swellings underneath the frontal lobes. It is the only sense that has such a direct physical connection to the brain. Every two to four weeks, the olfactory cells are replenished by stem cells. With the onset of dementia, the sense of smell is the first to suffer.

There is currently a patent, by researchers from Columbia University lead by Davangere Devanand, for a test using scents that include cheese, clove, fruit punch, leather, lemon, lilac, lime, menthol, orange, pineapple, smoke and strawberry. Using this test, the clinicians can predict that an individual who cannot recognize three of the ten scents are five times more likely to develop Alzheimer's disease. It has also been found to predict Parkinson's disease as well as certain types of schizophrenia and brain tumors. There are some sixty-seven medical conditions identified as possibly causing loss of smell—dementia being one of them. Some of these causes are temporary, such as colds, and nasal allergies such as hay fever. It may also occur due to some medications and localized nasal polyps and tumors. Such factors reduce the odds of making the patent smell test a very reliable indicator in predicting dementia.

It is likely however, that if we have depleted our stem cell reserve to enable us to replace our olfactory epithelium cells, then there will be other serious repercussions. This loss of stem cells eventually affects the maintenance of the neurons in the brain. If dementia is the result of stem cell depletion, then logically the first sign is the loss of smell, since the turnover of olfactory cells occurs so quickly. The loss of stem cells causing dementia would also explain how the disease progresses. Neural stem cells in the adult brain are located specifically–but not limited to–the subventricular zone that surrounds the main pocket of fluid-filled cavities inside each side of the brain and the dentate gyrus of the hippocampal formation. Early in the disease, dementia patients start showing significantly smaller volumes of the right and the left hippocampus and the left frontal lobe compared to controls. These reductions correlate closely to the locations of where the concentration of stems cells is in the brain.

Stem cells offer a new portal for investigation. Researchers are looking at how normal cells can become stem cells, or how stem cells can be differentiated. The research findings are generating great interest, funding, and Nobel prizes. But an alternate way to stop aging involves the aging cells themselves. If we cannot control the telomeres, or provide enough replacement cells through stem cells, then why not fix the cells themselves.

Mitochondrial Dysfunction

In our body, most of our cells have a nucleus surrounded by a membrane. These cells are known as eukaryotic cells to differentiate them from prokaryotic cells that do not have a membrane. Eukaryotic cells serve as a complex factory of activity that include particular alien small organs called mitochondria. Mitochondria are a type of bacteria that the cell hosts, and it generates all the power for the cell. Having its own genetic material, separate from the cell's DNA, mitochondria converts the energy of food into small packets of energy batteries—called Adenosine TriPhosphate (ATP). These small battery packs power all of the cell's functions. Eukaryotic cells are everywhere in the body, and mitochondria exists in each one of them (sometimes cells have multiple mitochondria). When the mitochondria malfunction, a wide range of disorders ensues. Symptoms in older adults include loss of muscle coordination, muscle weakness, visual problems, hearing problems, learning disabilities, heart disease, liver disease, kidney disease, gastrointestinal disorders, respiratory disorders, neurological problems (including dementia), autonomic dysfunction (causing dizziness and fainting and not being able to control heart rate. It remains a puzzle why these mitochondria die–we simply call it senescence (cell death). Surely cell death is not good for longevity—it is truly a death switch. Our search for a switch, for binary answers is yet again deflected by the nuance of how the body orchestrates life. There is a new twist to this story.

Cellular Senescence

Although a feature of aging is a gradual loss of function that starts at the molecular and cellular level, cell death is not easy to understand. The death of cells—known as senescence—initiates a cascade of events that are not completely understood.

In 2013 Mekayla Storer, and her colleagues in Barcelona, and Daniel Muñoz-Espín, and his colleagues in Madrid, published some interesting conjectures on this theme. When a cell dies, it was always assumed that it is in response to age, stress or trauma. In fact, the anti-aging industry is built upon the foundation of stopping cell death with the hope of making us immortal. But these Spanish researchers have shown that cell death is a necessary process for development. That in order for other cells to grow they need some of the cells to die first and create a pattern. This study, uniquely, comes not from samples of older adults but from embryos.

For the first time, evidence exists showing that cell death is programmed in order for specific organs to be able to develop. Cell death is not only a part of development but is a required part it. These cells are like an advance reconnaissance party that charts out a territory and by dying, send out directions for the main party to follow (or not). In the embryo, when a cell dies, its death instructs new tissue growth. The necessity of cell death has been shown to help control normal limb formation, nervous system development, development of kidneys and ear formation.

These studies show that cell death is a necessary part of development of normal organs. This is new insights into our biology. Such studies are a death knell to the anti-aging industry. Cell death is a necessary process in order to pave the way for new cells to grow, which enables the growth of different parts of our bodies.

The process is determined by how the dead cells are cleaned by specialized cells, with new cells following this track. When cells do not die, then problems with development result. It is no wonder that birth defects are in parts of the embryos prone to dysfunction in this process. The death of cells and how they are cleaned up is instrumental for the normal growth of cells. Such a system of rejuvenation is important for older adults because dying cells and how they are cleaned up have complementary functions in cancer. We do not know the exact relationship (whether one encourages the other or not) but we know they are related because we can listen to them communicating.

Cells communicate in short distances—known as paracrine—and long distances—through hormones and endocrine system. This language could be what differentiates good dying cells from bad dying cells—cancer. Good dying cells have a different short distance message from cancer cells. Good dying cells might call out to the cleaner cells while cancer cells give short messages that keep the cleaner cells away. How these two different types of dying cells work in aging is still unknown, but we now know that cell death communicates with living cells. Cellular death is therefore a re-addressing of a balance and can have either beneficial or deleterious effects on its neighbors.

Conclusion of Search for the Switch

The fountain of youth construct is the main narrative in the biology of immortality. The folklore of reversing aging remains an ambition for some scientists. But reversing aging is not science, since science remains blind to outcomes. Science is a method of looking for answers. It is not a method for achieving specific result that is the role of applied science. Instead, science is a method, a way of understanding reality, a manner of studying it.

The main narrative pervading immortality studies ignores the fact that aging is not all negative. The same narrative that we uncovered when examining how genes promote longevity applies to the biology of aging–that a body is not an island but is intimately and inextricably connected to the environment. Within this general observation, we can succinctly summarize theories of the biology of aging as a series of survival strategies in addressing changing environmental conditions. The use of supplements is at best aiding this process and at worst, toxic. Many behaviors can promote longevity–not smoking, being active, eating quality foods, sleeping well, de-stressing: all are beneficial. But by themselves, these strategies simply protect us from causing harm.

Our lifespan is set and living healthy will ensure that we reach it, not that we will escape it. The search for the fountain of youth, translated in the modern age through the promotion of supplements is a continuation of the myth. Some of these supplements might promote health. But to understand how that is possible, we need to move beyond the Caloric Restriction and Anti-Oxidant hypothesis and look at the multiple switches that may exist.

A hierarchy of biological processes exists. From the simple mitochondria, an organelle within cells, to the genetic material contained in our DNA, there is evidence of coordination. Each component relies on other components in this biological house of cards.

Although the story of the many switches involved in aging remains to be told, there is unlikely to be a panacea, a single solution. Research will continue to build up the puzzle, until we get a better picture of it. That is the method of science. But our psychology is different. And our quest for immortality continues to expose the conflict between our desire to learn and the desire to "cure" aging and gain immortality.

————————∞————————

Chapter 4

Survival Package: Balance

Let there be spaces in your togetherness, And let the winds of the heavens dance between you. Love one another but make not a bond of love: Let it rather be a moving sea between the shores of your souls. Fill each other's cup but drink not from one cup. Give one another of your bread but eat not from the same loaf. Sing and dance together and be joyous, but let each one of you be alone, Even as the strings of a lute are alone though they quiver with the same music.

– Kahlil Gibran (1923) *The Prophet*. A Borzoi Book.

C an we know how the body ages by looking at individual components? As we progress with this story of immortality we are appreciating the limitations of each individual component in explaining the whole. The analogy is looking at people dancing without being able to hear the music. We can guess what is happening but it is the music that provides the meaning and our understanding of the whole. In order to be able to understand why we age, we have to take a broader view of what our bodies really encompass. To do that, we have to start outside of our body.

We are more bacteria than human. Our predominant biology is composed of alien cells. And this expansion of "us" also needs to include our environment. Many processes operate in equilibrium in our body, which is a virtual orchestra of events. Not one switch, or multiple switches control this process. Accordingly, the story to find a switch has ended with a much broader concept of who we are as human. And when we look at the body and the mind we find that we are more of a colony than an entity.

Bacteria Colonizers

Although it is usually estimated that there are ten times more bacterial cells than human cells in your body, in 2013, the American Academy of Microbiology suggested that the real figure is probably closer to three bacterial cells for each human cell. This conservative estimate still adds up to 111 trillion bacterial cells in our body. Although smaller than human cells, and weighing only 1-3% of our body weight, the 500-1,000 species of bacteria that inhabit our body have evolved with us for millions of years. With each of us, this world of microbes has accompanied us since inception. They colonized us from the start.

Andrew Moeller, from the University of California, Berkeley, and his colleagues while studying human gut bacteria found that just as humans share common ancestors our gut bacteria also share common ancestors with the microbes that apes carry. Gut bacteria therefore are not simply acquired from the environment, but have coevolved with us humans for millions of years. They have evolved to help shape our immune systems and development. Bacteria are used for signaling, cellular differentiation, and cell death, as well as maintaining control of the cell cycle and cell growth. As we have seen in the previous chapter, even how each individual cell in our bodies generates energy is determined by mitochondria. The presence of these organelles varies from one per cell to more than 2000 in liver cells. Without mitochondria, we will not function. Mitochondria generate the energy we need for the cell to function. It is humbling to learn that such an integrate part of our existence, mitochondria, have their own genetic code and replicate independent of the rest of our cells. They consist of bacteria that were absorbed into our cells and now form an integral relationship with human cells—an endosymbiotic relationship in our body. However, unlike this synergetic relationship, some bacteria stay in our body as independent contractors.

As independent contractors, bacteria reside all over our body—inside and out—we see its importance primarily in maintaining balance in the human gut. Fewer physical changes occur in older adults' gastric system than any other system in the body. Although the stomach loses its elasticity and might be more prone to damage—primarily as a result of medications—the small and large intestine, pancreas, liver, and gallbladder change minimally with age. As a result of this consistency, the changes that evolve inside our gut are argued to come from bacteria that inhabit this internal world.

The 100 trillion microorganisms in our stomach engage in fermenting, killing off other harmful bacteria and viruses, enhancing our immune system and producing vitamins and hormones. This bacterial activity is so necessary to the body that their outcome functions as an independent organ—a virtual, "forgotten" organ. Here, bacteria help extract energy and nutrients from our food. This sharing of benefits shows in experiments where bacteria-free rodents have to consume nearly a third more calories than normal rodents to maintain their body weight. Less well understood is the role of fungi and protozoa, which also inhabit this hidden world in our gut.

In 2012, Marcus Claesson and Ian Jeffery from University College Cork in Ireland and their colleagues reported this bacterial world in our gut changes among some older adults. They argue that these changes in the type of bacteria lead to frailty and mortality. Claesson found that institutionalized older adults have different bacteria in their gut—as a result of a restricted diet—causing them to becoming physically weaker. Martin Blaser from New York University and Glenn Webb from Vanderbilt University went further when they tried to explain how bacteria kill older adults. In 2014 Blaser and Webb argued that modern medical problems, such as inflammation-induced early cancer, resistance to infectious diseases and degenerative diseases, are in response to change in the bacteria composition, as we get older. This revelation is startling enough, but the authors argue that such terminal bacteria have an evolutionary cause. Using mathematical models the authors show how bacteria evolved because they contributed to the stability of early human populations: Enhancing the survivability of younger adults while increasing vulnerability of older adults. Such an evolutionary process has advantages, but the authors argue that in the modern world bacteria's legacy has become a burden on human longevity.

Such a conjecture is not as fanciful as it might initially seem and we will revisit this concept later on in this book.

The idea that bacteria are not just passive guests is further supported by evidence that shows how they control day-to-day activities. Sometimes bacteria call for delivery.

Gut microbes can produce neurotransmitters that alter your mood, and even may control your appetite. These cause you to crave food that bacteria enjoy but which might be detrimental to your overall health. Such risky behaviors, in some cases, cause disease and early death. An infection of a parasite called Toxoplasma gondii, for example, makes rats attracted to cats. Since the bacteria can reproduce only in cats (their vector, how they transmit to other animals and multiply) they make rats lethargic around cats improving the chances of the rat being caught and improving the bacteria's chances of infecting the cat and reproducing.

In humans, the same microbe increases the chance they will suffer from schizophrenia or suicidal depression. Bacteria are necessary in balancing the biological activities in our human body. In one example scientists are using bacteria that cause botulism to eradicate tumors. In another, Linlin Guo and her colleagues from the Buck Institute for Research on Aging have increased lifespan in flies by altering bacteria in their intestine. It seems that bacteria form an important system in the body that might have repercussions on our longevity. Our body is a universe of organic activity, and we are still learning about this internal miracle. How it is maintained remains unknown.

The concept that our body is a constellation of many other organisms that depend on us and we depend on them ushers an exciting concept in biology. But it makes the search for a binary simple answer to the cause of longevity that much more complicated. In addition, bacteria are not the only alien organisms in our bodies. While we are in the womb, cells pass between twins or triplets and sometimes from previous siblings that occupied the womb. Around one in twelve non-identical twins and one in five triplets, for example, have not one, but two blood groups: one produced by their own cells, and one absorbed from their twin. There are even anecdotal examples, where a mother passed on her twin sister's genes, and not her own, to her children. The process of separating her DNA into eggs (meiosis) allowed for her twin sister's genes to be carried in her eggs to be different from genes in the rest of her body. This makes Kin Selection a biological and not just a social phenomenon.

Alternatively, cells from an older sibling might stay around the mother's body, only to find their way into your body after you are conceived. Lee Nelson from the University of Washington is examining whether cells from the mother herself may be implanted in the baby's brain and the other way around, where a baby's genetic material finds itself in the mother's brain. Nelson took slices of women's brain tissue and screened their genome for signs of the Y-chromosome (the chromosome that determines male characteristics). More than half of mothers had Y-chromosome male cells in multiple brain regions. The authors cite an observation showing that these alien cells seemed to decrease the chances that the mother would subsequently develop Alzheimer's disease—though exactly why remains a mystery.

Our body is home to a universe of external biological entities. If we perceive our body as a constellation of organisms interfacing with the environment, then we see that the scope of our biology broadens. The idea that we have biological permeability to the environment radially changes out view of humans as a closed entity. Not only does our body hosts other organisms and blends-in with the environment, our brain is similarly influenced by external conditions, both in terms of how it functions and how it behaves.

Mirror Neurons

Some specialized areas in our brain "mirror" our environment. In the 1980s, the Italian Giacomo Rizzolatti and his colleagues at the University of Parma, first observed mirror neurons in monkeys. Although mirror neurons exist in most animals, in humans they have been observed in multiple areas of the brain, with as many as 10 percent of neural cells devoted to mirroring. A mirror neuron fires both when a person acts and also while observing the same action performed by another person. We learn by looking. Such mirror neurons respond directly to what is observed in the environment. Our brain responds and mimics the activation of another person's behavior and activity.

Both the existence of alien cells and mirror neurons highlight how susceptible we are to our environment. Although we perceive ourselves as a separate entity, our immediate environment constantly influences both our body and mind. This observation is radical. Our permeable life cannot be managed without modifying our environment.

A history exists between our environment and us and is likely to have started early on in our development. There must be an optimum time for the environment, especially bacteria, to influence our development in anticipation of the environmental demands that will be placed upon the body. Such a theory has emerged that argues that environmental conditions determine, to some degree, our health and longevity. This influence occurs even before we are born.

Interacting with the environment

Your mother helped you prepare for the outside world while you were still in her womb. Not just through contributing to half your genes, her nourishment and warmth, but also by passing on her body's bacterial, fungal, and viral colonizers. We know that these alien inhabitants play a role in our overall health, but they also determine the first message about the type of environment that you will meet when you are born. Mothers impart all this bacteria to the yet unborn child. It is a very specific environment–no two mothers are the same. The mother herself is sampling and selecting bacteria to transfer to her fetus.

Each birth is unique in terms of the bacteria transmitted. By transmitting these alien colonizers, the mother begins training her child's immunity to prepare for the life outside. Although most people now know about vaginal bacteria and the importance of vaginal birth in contrast to caesarian birth for promoting good bacteria in the baby, the baby's bacteria in uterus is already different from its mother.. The birthing process, then, would be the second stop on a tour of the maternal infection with microbes.

Once on the outside, a baby's first embrace with his mother transfers her skin microbiome—the bacterial aura that surrounds us. After this exchange, then there is the exposure to our mother's breast milk. This creamy bacterial cocktail is an individualized inoculation composed of over 700 types of bacteria. For the production of milk, bacteria inside the mother is collected and transported around the body using the lymphatic system that converge in our groin, arm pits, and among lactating women, their breasts. At the instant of birth, we are showered with thousands of different kinds of bacteria. Our first breath, our first food, our first touch is an exchange of bacteria. Our environment is saying, "welcome".

And this world of small biological entities—microbiome—exists inside as well as all over the outside of our bodies and our immediate environment. A baby already exists as a micro-universe, made up of more than 1,000 different bacterial species comprising 3.3 million unique genes—150 times more genes than in the human genome. Although the gut has the most obvious concentration, and hence the most research, all parts of the body function as a host to these alien microbes that have colonized us for millennia.

As adults, we also share bacteria with other people—not just during intimate moments, but also when we interact in close proximity. An aura of bacteria and micro-organisms As a doctoral researcher with Oregon State University, James Meadow and his colleagues published a study that examined the unique qualities of this microbiotic plume that extends a few meters around individuals. Each plume has a distinct signature that identifies you. We exude and share these airborne micro-organisms with others, and others share theirs with us. We start to see a less distinct biological presence of self. The environment becomes very much blurred within us, and with us blurring into the environment.

Micro-organisms also exist within buildings and the geography that we live in. These microbes are specific to the place; home, office, public venues, parks. We do not know their exact significance but they must influence us in some way. The significance of geography—and the biological and emotional relationship we have with it—is when we find clusters of extremely long-lived individuals identified in the Blue Zones that have lived in places that were (in the past) secluded from others and they did not travel out of their community. The geography they live in remains secluded from the outside world, and they tend not to travel. This has beneficial social and biological consequences.

When one colony of bacteria determines the colony on another part of our body, it creates a balance and to create this balance there has to be communication among these different colonies. This communication is known as the metabolomic system. Since metabolomics involves all the small molecules in our body, it allows us to listen in on how these microbes communicate, perhaps shining some light on the cause of diseases and how genes are expressed. So far, causality has been difficult to prove between microbes and disease, unless we understand the mechanism that the metabolomics system can provide. Microbiomes and metabolomes of infants with asthma and allergies had deficiencies of several native bacterial species in the gut. Interestingly, these asthmatic children also displayed high concentrations of pro-inflammatory T-cells and relatively low concentrations of T cells that protect against asthma and allergy. Autism showed an elevation in the concentration of two bacterial species in the gut. Some emerging studies are exposing the relationship complex diseases have with our microbiome. But we are at the early stages of accepting that our biology as humans includes other alien micro-organisms.

Understanding the language of these colonies will clarify the roles this alien universe has on our health and longevity. First, the skin acts as a constant thermometer of the outside world—a permeable barrier that hosts the most varied colonies of bacteria. Patterns and organizations exist within these separate clusters—they are not a random splattering of bacteria. This is a functional colony, an entity.

After the skin, the first ingestion of the environment starts in the mouth. In 2010, microbiologist Floyd Dewhirst with Forsyth Institute in Cambridge, Massachusetts, and his colleagues identified some 700 different microbes that inhabit the human mouth. And these colonies are organized in a very hierarchical manner. The microbes not only infect the mouth and the teeth, but they can easily slide from the mouth through the windpipe into the stomach, or become airborne and sucked into the lungs.

Oral bacteria have also been shown to cause cardiovascular disease, some cancer, including pancreatic and colorectal cancer, and rheumatoid arthritis. Among pregnant women bacteria in the mouth also influences the microbiome in the placenta affecting the unborn child directly. In some cases, oral bacteria have also been linked to preterm birth.

A constant flow of bacteria is evident, back and forth from the air and the mouth and air passage into the lungs and back out again. The lung microbiome, although less rich, is nevertheless important. Studies now link lung microbiome to chronic diseases, such as cystic fibrosis and chronic obstructive pulmonary disease. More direct action from bacteria have been found in relation to Chlamydia and bacteria in the penis that create chemical conditions that prevent the infection. That the male penis microbiome might be synchronized with his partner's microbiome extends the influence other people have on our bodies.

Interestingly, the ethnicity of a woman determines the vaginal microbiome, as well as its alkaline-acidity level. The composition can change within a day and after biological events such as menopause and most significantly during pregnancy. In addition to introducing microbes to populate her infant's gut, a mother's microbiome during pregnancy and lactation appears to affect her own health. Changes in the gut microbiome during pregnancy correlate with gains in fat and reduction in insulin sensitivity.

Jumping Genes

Bacteria appear to be perfectly adapted to a variety of environments. There are so many types of bacteria that there seems to be the right bacteria for whatever environment it encounters. The question is how these bacteria interact with humans.

Bacteria respond by employing elegant mechanisms. While most cells—eukaryotes—have two or more chromosomes, bacteria possess a single looped chromosome. Looped chromosomes, because they are circular, are immortal since there are no end bits—telomeres—that shorten and unravel the chromosome when they replicate. Many bacteria, including some yeasts and fungi, possess additional genes–bits of genes that float around in the body of the cell. These foreign looped bits of DNA, are also immortal and replicate by themselves. In 1952 Joshua Lederberg named these bits of floating DNA "Plasmids."

Plasmids are simple DNA with fewer than 30 genes that replicate independently of the host bacteria. While plasmids are not essential to the survival of the host bacteria, they make unique contribution to their host. Not only do they respond quickly to environmental stress, for example, by generating anti-bodies, they also have the ability to move out of the host bacteria into other bacteria or into humans. They can move horizontally between bacteria and into humans—horizontal gene transfer. Studying the transfer of plasmids has revolutionized our understanding of genetics.

Joshua Lederberg and his assistants at the University of Wisconsin identified three methods by which plasmids transfer their DNA to other bacteria or to human cells. This is not a passive process—both push and pull factors come into play. The host seems to want these bits of DNA. We are not sure of the exact mechanism. We know that it happens but we do not fully understand nor how or why. Exchange occurs among the plasmids themselves (Conjugation), or when dead bacteria release their plasmids—which are then absorbed and incorporate by other bacteria (Transformation) and lastly where viruses or bacteria can act as vehicles to transfer genes into humans (Transduction).

Although it was always assumed that genes can only be transferred vertically from parent to offspring, these little circular DNA molecules continue to teach us about a whole new world. Horizontal gene transfer seems to be more common than we assumed. In the fetus, cells pass between twins or triplets and sometimes from previous siblings that occupied the womb. Around one in twelve non-identical twins and one in five of triplets, for example, have not one, but two blood groups: one produced by their own cells, and one absorbed from their twin. There are even examples where a mother passed on her twin sister's genes, and not her own, to her children. Her eggs carried different genes from the rest of the body. Alternatively, cells from an older sibling might stay around the mother's body, only to find their way into your body after you are conceived. These observations provide one simple lesson of how permeable our genetic material is to people that are family: our kin. Lee Nelson from the University of Washington is examining whether cells from the mother herself may be implanted in the baby's brain and also to reciprocate, where a baby's genetic material finds itself in the mother's brain. Nelson took slices of women's brain tissue and screened their genome for signs of the Y-chromosome—the male sex chromosome. More than half of mothers had Y-chromosome male cells in multiple brain regions. The authors cite a correlational observation showing that these alien cells seemed to decrease the chances that the mother would subsequently develop Alzheimer's disease—although exactly why remains a mystery. Many such mysteries still remain to be uncovered, and answers still to be pursued. The deeper we search the more social the answers become. Even in the depths of the brain, we find social influences that are far stronger than the intermixing of genes with your siblings or children.

Horizontal gene transfer also works with plasmids that can unload their gene content across species, and in particular insert their gene into our DNA. This "infective heredity" happens all the time. And not surprisingly, the older we get the more likely it becomes that we gain more of these alien genes.

Infective heredity

The best candidate for humans to receive alien genes is through plasmids within bacteria. We have an incredible variety of bacteria both inside and outside the human body. Numerous studies now show that our human genome has historically acquired numerous genes via horizontal transfer from bacteria, viruses and archae—single cell micro-organisms. All life on Earth can be grouped into three main groups: Eukaryota, Archaea and Bacteria. Genes from all these groups have been contributing to our human adaptive evolution and such contributions are encouraged by nature.

But how do plasmids know where they need to be on the chromosome? Insight into this part of the dance came about with "jumping genes," known as transposons. These segments of DNA move about within the chromosome and establish new genetic sequences. First discovered by Barbara McClintock in the 1940s, transposons behave somewhat like plasmids—except that these jumping genes can be from the same host. Barbara McClintock's work was revolutionary in that she suggested that these "jumping genes" change places along chromosomes. Even when these bacterial genes have become human, so to speak, they move around the chromosome to find the best fit. Sometimes they even jump across to other chromosomes within the same genome. In their new position, these genes have a different and more utilitarian function.

In the 1940s and 50s this idea was met with "puzzlement, even hostility" from the scientific community. But by 1983 McClintock's work was recognized for its brilliance, and she was awarded the Nobel Prize for medicine. McClintock was the first American woman to win a Nobel Prize without sharing it with anyone else. Her work provided evidence that the composition of our genes—our genome—changes while we are living. The longer we live before having children, the more likely that these new genetic improvements are transmitted to our children. So now we have figured out the method of how Michael Rose's flies create a time stamp on their genes. Plasmids, especially transposons are at work throughout the aging process. Your genetic contribution matures–a clever system if your progeny needs to be prepared to mature and transfer their genes at older ages. This system of gene modification is an excellent way of responding to the environment and transferring this knowledge to your children.

Subsequently we have found other mechanisms where genes rearrange themselves throughout our lives. Such insights diminish the rigid genetic interpretation put forward by the father of genetics, Gregor Mendel. In one sense our genes are modular. Our chromosomes seem to be able to mix and match genes depending on the environmental needs imposed upon us. Barbara McClintock was also the first scientist to correctly speculate on the basic concept of epigenetics—how some genes can be switched on and off—changing what a gene does without changing the composition of the chromosome. She predicted that we have a genetic amplifier: some genes can be subdued while other genes are promoted.

Unlike evolution via gene duplications and mutations–a slow and incremental process–horizontal gene transfer and epigenetics point to new genes and different amplification of the influence of genes. These two methods of gene enhancement permit humans to acquire fast response to environmental challenges, clearly an important ability in order for a species to adapt and survive. In 1999 the UCLA researchers Ravi Jain, Maria. Rivera, and James Lake tested whether this transfer of genes is continuous or occurred at one time in our evolutionary past. They found that horizontal gene transfer happens continuously. As you read this, your genes are in a state of flux, acquiring new adaptive features. The authors further argue that horizontal transfer has been an important factor in the evolution of our genes. Although such horizontal transfer contributes only a few percentage of our whole collection of genes, nevertheless these transfers are significant. These new plasmid additions directly address new environmental conditions. Without such genetic modifications, we will be less resilient to the new environmental stressors imposed upon us.

This is a valuable lesson–that our environment is much more important for our biology, and therefore for aging, than we initially assumed. We need to re-examine who we mean by "us". We seem to be a colony rather than an entity, and our genes—which in the past were assumed to be immutable laws etched in stone—are rather computer codes not only from our parents, maybe our siblings who shred our mother's womb, but also from plasmids (among others). For aging, the implications of this continuous interaction are enormous.

A number of explanations in biology compete to explain of how aging occurs. Most explanations focus on cell senescence (cell death.) We have looked at some of the genetic theories; Telomere attrition, epigenetic alterations and genomic instability. The genetic theories rely on mistakes that accumulate in older age. With increasing age, the copies that we make of each cell will have more imperfections. The analogy is of photocopying a picture, then taking that copy and making another copy from it, and so on. Eventually imperfections are introduced, accumulate and further reproduced. Other, complementary explanations, range from the effect of cellular activity, to coordination of proteins, the decline in generating energy in the cell (mitochondria malfunctions), the depletion of stem cells that can replace damaged cells, reduced communication among cells, and programmed cell death (telomeres). We need to understand each of these explanations to understand the symphony playing in our body/mind.

We have yet to determine how caloric restriction and anti-oxidants extend longevity in humans. It is difficult to conduct diet-controlled, randomized, long-term survival studies due to compliance, cost, complexity and ethical issues. Piper Hunt with the National Instates of Health and his colleagues in 2011 suggested that multiple ways exist for increasing lifespan in the roundworm, using methods that include oxidative stress, thermal stress, and even pesticide.

These explorations illustrate the tantalizing realization that there might be "multiple switches" that can be turned on or off, through a variety of short shocks, to induce a long lasting biological reaction. One of those reactions is increased longevity.

It seems that a wide variety of shocks can act to induce a positive reaction. As early as 1956, Charles E Murry with the University of Washington called this preconditioning–where a prior less severe stress (e.g., mild heart attack) affords protection against a subsequent and more severe challenging exposure/dose (e.g., massive heart attack). It seems that because hormesis can be induced by so many seemingly negative conditions, and because the effects are long lasting, hormesis could be one of the mechanisms that maintains our survival package and controls the switch for our mortality/longevity.

Hormesis

Diagram 2: A Selection of Individual Supplements and Possible Mechanisms for Improved Longevity and their relationship to Hormesis.

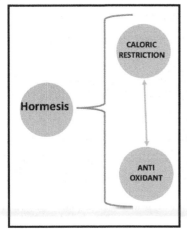

The overarching mechanism for maintaining health and longevity for the long term is likely hermetic change. As many possible contributing mechanisms promote longevity, the "switch" that can engage many of these mechanisms may be hormesis. At this stage, very little information exists on such an overarching and coordinating mechanism. Research focuses on individual mechanisms. But more recent understanding suggests a broad array of cell responses to low-level shocks might have long-term consequences. The body responds in radical ways, including the increased production of chemicals and proteins that protect cells, the production of restorative proteins and hormones capable of stimulating cellular health, long proteins that have preventative and protective effects against errant cells and free radicals, and protein chaperones that help other proteins form and behave as desired. How such oversight is coordinated within our body remains an enigma.

Hormesis represents a gyroscope in maintaining a balance between an individual and the environment. Even if a slight elevation of a certain toxic chemical, event or condition in the environment occurs, the body chemistry changes to prepare for it. But this balancing act is not without limitation. The capacity for the body to make biological/chemical adjustments is limited, but there is plasticity in this system of person–environment interaction. Nadine Saul with the Humboldt-University of Berlin and his colleagues have argued that the process of hormesis is a balance that has both positive and negative outcomes. It emerged that for every longevity improvement, there is a reduction in the capacity of the organism for growth, mobility, stress resistance, or reproduction. Saul argues (correctly it seems) that longevity comes at a price, and although hormesis seems to promote longevity, other hormetic costs may ensue, some of which are unknown and unpredictable.

The concept of hormesis has a long history. As early as 1493, Theophrastus Bombastus von Hohenheim a Swiss pharmacist identified the concept that "the dose makes the poison." In the mid 1880s, Hugo Schulz, a German pharmacologist was looking for an alternative disinfectant to carbolic acid. While evaluating the effect of multiple chemicals on yeast, Schulz observed that at low concentrations, some chemicals promoted yeast while at higher concentrations it killed the yeast off. At the time, medicine ignored Schulz' observations, burying both the finding and Schulz's career.   Chester Southam first mentioned Hormesis in his 1941 University of Idaho undergraduate thesis (page 23). The observation usually ascribed to another later paper in 1943 when Southam, then a master student working with his supervisor John Ehrlich, wrote his thesis on fungi in trees. Hormesis explains how exposure to low levels of a known toxin confers resistance or resilience. What does not kill you make you stronger. When getting a vaccine, we use the hermetic principle of getting the body to react and become stronger against a low-level toxin (virus). Revived again in 1980 by Thomas Luckey of the University of Missouri, some lasting impressions resulted in the publication of *Ionizing Radiation and Hormesis.*

The mechanism of hormesis remains an enigma, although we continue to learn more about how the body develops resilience in response to changes in the environment. In 1962, Italian geneticist Ferruccio Ritossa discovered that heat shock proteins are produced when cells are exposed to a variety of stresses. Initially identified with fruit flies that were exposed to a burst of heat resulting in the production of new proteins that help cells survive. The epigenes responsible for this are called "vitagenes" and maintain balance within cells under stressful conditions. As with the heat shock proteins, these act as chaperones, as minders, in assisting the establishment of "proper protein behavior." Despite these terms, we do not know how this function is carried out.

Similarly, we now acknowledge that caloric restriction itself might be effective because of its hermetic qualities—a shock to the body—rather than through diet. This might be the case since multiple ways exist for producing the same effect without adhering to a diet of calorie reduction. The underlying mechanism—rather than the reduction of calories—becomes important. And the underlying mechanism is a shock. If we accept this mechanism, then we should ask "why?" Why does a shock cause the body to build resilience?

The answer is both simple and radical, because the body is designed to do exactly that. In order for the body to accomplish this there must be some plasticity, some wiggle room. And our biology is a constellation of different entities that depend on each other. How it does this adaptation is more enigmatic, but we now know that there are plasmids and bacteria that help address the needs of our body. These might even recombine with our own DNA to make these adaptations more permanent.

The more we explore body the more we see that we are made up of collective alien organisms. In addition to genes that we inherit (in most cases, but not always) from both our parents, there are viruses, bacteria and potentially, other human cells within our body. And then there is the interpretation of these genes. Under certain conditions, some of these genes are amplified while others are muted. How such a system can be achieved is the story of epigenetics.

Epigenetics

Living in poor and dangerous neighborhoods has a direct effect on our hormones and stress chemicals—such as interleukin 6, which acts as both a pro-inflammatory cell signaling (cytokine) and an anti-inflammatory muscle protein (myokine) that indicates body stress. A stressful environment—such as poor neighborhood—results in negative changes in the chemical composition of older adults, regardless of other factors. These chemicals initiate longer lasting changes in the body because they switch on and off the expression of some genes. These epi-genes ("epi" meaning above genes) can be switched on and off in order to help establish and maintain a consistent optimum level of chemical balance within the body. Environmental factors such as mercury in water, second-hand smoke, diet including foliate, pharmaceuticals, pesticides, air pollutants, industrial chemicals, heavy metals, hormones in water, nutrition, and behavior have been shown to affect epigenetics. Further, epi-genetic changes are associated with specific outcomes such as cancer, diabetes, obesity, infertility, respiratory diseases, allergies, and neurodegenerative disorders such as Parkinson's and Alzheimer's diseases. Our body changes our epi-genes—establishing an optimum level of chemical balance—in response to our environment and which influence our overall health.

Diagram 3: Possible Mechanisms of Interaction Allowing Human vs. Environment Adaptation.

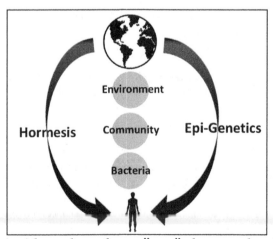

Accumulating evidence suggests that the body serves as a meeting place of interaction, a venue with the outside world—its geography, the community, and significant others. Accepting that there is not just a "me" inside us but also a "we," then we begin to better understand how the environment—community, family and friends—can determine our health outcomes. How all these influences come together remains a conundrum. Because proteins are the main building blocks in life, one of the avenues for exploring the construct of balance in the body is to understand the balance in protein synthesis and maintenance.

Loss of Proteostasis

Proteostasis refers to protein homeostasis—the balance that exists in the choreographed dance of manufacturing and distributing proteins around the body. Proteins—which are made up of amino acids—function as enzymes, hormones and body tissues. The importance of proteins is expressed by the recent ambition to map all human proteins through the Human Proteome Project. That we mapped the genome—the location of all genes—does not mean very much if we do not know what those codes mean. The role of genes is to encode and manufacture proteins.

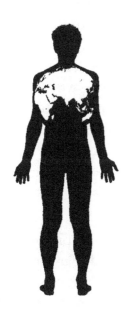

Proteins and everything involved in the production—reading the code, creating the mechanism to produce protein, selecting amino acids in sequence to build specific proteins, checking the integrity of each protein molecule sequence, folding them, monitoring and then recycling them when they are no longer useful—are what genes are all about. This includes Deregulated Nutrient-Sensing. Within each cell resides the mechanism that identifies the protein it requires. With an ever-changing environment, a fast and efficient response is crucial for survival. Cells have evolved mechanisms that sense nutrient concentrations—for example glucose and cholesterol—and quickly respond to any changing needs. Sometimes this sensing mechanism malfunctions and the cells do not respond, or do not respond fast enough, resulting in metabolic diseases (e.g., Type 2 diabetes).

We do not know the whole story of proteins. Scientists make simplified determinations despite knowing only a very small proportion of the biology of cell functioning. We might have traced most of the dance moves, but we still do not know the music that proteins are dancing to. That symphony that all our cells are all dancing to remains silent in our investigations. With a complex choreography of steps, there also remain new ones to identify. We are missing the poetry because of the words, and we are missing the music because of the steps. In older adults (and some diseases) this choreography becomes disturbed. The main cause of this disruption is thought to be the effect of oxidation through Reactive Oxygen Species-ROS, as discussed in earlier chapter. But we do not really know. We are listening to silence when we try and understand this whole process and how it becomes unbalanced. We know how certain biological pathways affect the balance, but we do not know the overall mechanism. We see the end result–the accumulation of disorderly proteins.

Conclusion searching for balance

Overall, the search for a balance in our biology has taken us on a wondrous magic carpet ride around the intricacies of biology and the very intimate relationship we have with our environment. The more details we accumulate in our knowledge of the biology aging, the more apparent our relationship with the environment becomes central to our survival. Although we know a lot about the mechanisms of our biology, our understanding has two stark omissions. First, our knowledge is uneven. We seem to know a lot about certain biological processes (chemical reactions in cells) but very little about others (senescence in fetuses). Secondly, we still do not understand how all of our biology is coordinated. What symphony is being played? These two blind spots result in science looking at specific biological mechanism distinctly separate from the environment. But this is slowly changing. The continuing exploration of protein behavior and how organs communicate with each other through paracrine signaling (short-distance communication) and hormones (long distance communication) highlights the importance of maintaining balance for the body. The emerging emphasis on Proteostasis–protein homeostasis–the balance that exists in the choreographed dance of manufacturing and distributing proteins around the body—holds great promise in elucidating the role of the environment, both internal and external, in maintaining life. The ultimate survival method for genes is to ensure that we are matched with the unique and ever-changing environment that we find ourselves in. This is the true story of the biology of immortality.

Science is moving us away from the most tenacious folklore, that of the fountain of youth. Although the growing anti-aging business attracts advocates, the real science means staying away from applied pharmacology. We are more bacteria than human; our predominant biology is composed of alien cells. This expansion of "us" also needs to include our environment. We learned this valuable lesson in the preceding chapter on genetics. The same is true for our biology. Our environment is much more important for aging than we initially assumed. Plasmids interact with our genes and as much as a couple of percentages of our genes are alien genes. Our environment resides within our codes for humanity. We saw that especially with how the fetus is influenced by the environment–that if there is a mismatch between what the fetus is designed to expect and the reality when it is born, then negative consequences ensue. It seems that throughout the exploration of biology and immortality, an appreciation exists that there are gains and losses. Our biological plasticity—how much our bodies can accommodate change—determines the balance we maintain. A push for one attribute results in a reduction in another. Our biology is a balance. The implications for the study of the biology of immortality are definitive.

Increased longevity comes at a price. Although our bodies are designed to have some flexibility—biological plasticity—in responding to our immediate environment, it seems that there is a price for such modification. The role of hormesis, as the harbinger of a changing environment, exploits this biological plasticity. No fountain of youth can exist within this nuanced biological function. From inception through our growth in the womb, during our birth, and then through our development we have set the stage for our interaction with the environment and have determined our resilience to ill health. Longevity is an expression, and not a separate component of health. Our biology comprises a life-long symphony and we become products of our time. We are meant to die because that is our strategy in life. How long we live is determined by how we respond to our environment. A balance exists. But earlier biologists were also right about how certain diseases associated with age seem to flourish.

Genes that show up in aging—Huntington's, Alzheimer's disease, heart disease, and many others—are passed on to our children because they do not show up until much later in life. But this interpretation does not explain the advantage of having longer-lived relatives and kin. Is there an advantage for having these diseases? Whether it is antagonist pleiotropy—the concept that there might be advantageous features of the disease at early stages—or whether it is statistically significant or not. Regardless of the interpretation, the question is relevant. Nature is not hoodwinked into promoting old age with all its associated diseases. Mathematical models started to show greater predictive value when family was included. Unlike any other animal, we transfer wealth, capital and wisdom to successive generations. Gene survival needs to include the broader community, and the family (kin).

So far, we have identified that our package for survival includes living longer—thanks to a bigger brain. That longevity is somehow wired-in. Finding a switch for how longevity works has been elusive, although some processes are implicated. All the processes have one thing in common–they are sensitive to the environment. Earlier mathematical models show that the contribution older adults make to their family is one-sided. They miss the opportunity to highlight how the family and community contribute back to the older adult. Having a consistent extended family around you provides constancy in the lives of older people. And the best way to test this argument is to go to the masters of longevity themselves: Centenarians.

———————∞———————

Chapter 5

Lessons from Centenarians

There is nothing very remarkable about being immortal; with the exception of mankind, all creatures are immortal, for they know nothing of death. What is divine, terrible, and incomprehensible is to know oneself immortal.

Jorge Luis Borges (1998). *The Immortal Collected fictions (translated by Andrew Hurley)*. London: Penguin

Biblical belief holds that "our years are threescore years and ten; and if by reason of strength they be fourscore years, yet is their strength, labor and sorrow..." (Psalms 90:10). For those who have reached 100-year mark and have broken through the barrier of fourscore years (80 years), what is their strength, labor and sorrow? This chapter focuses on real life examples of extreme longevity. Nature has provided some exceptional examples.

Centenarians—those living to 100 years and beyond—are at the precipice of human longevity. Beyond them lies an unknown. In our continuing journey through immortality, they will henceforth be our guides. Luckily, incredible consistency exists among this group, which will help focus our exploration. The variance that we start seeing with older adults—referred to as heteroscedasticity—is partially removed among centenarians and to a greater extent among supercentenarians—those who live up to and beyond 110 years. Centenarians, in certain aspects, emerge as a uniquely homogeneous group. Not surprisingly, we find that centenarians have later onset of diseases–especially for supercentenarians, who only get diseases at the final stages before death. And then death comes quickly. On average, supercentenarians suffer five years of ill health before dying, whereas older adults spend an average of 17 years of ill health before dying. An observation that supports the expectation that with older death comes a reduction in the period of ill-health that proceeds it—known as the Compression of Morbidity.

The United States currently has the highest number of centenarians in the world, estimated at 72,197 in 2014. This statistic results partly from America's large population, California, the most populous state within the United States, similarly has the largest number of U.S. resident centenarians with 5,341. Despite recent inaccuracies in counting centenarians in Japan, where officials now say that they are unable to account for more than 1,000 of the country's 44,449 listed centenarians, Japan still has the highest percentage of centenarians. Most recent figures for 2015 show 61,568 Japanese centenarians. You are twice as likely to become a centenarian in Japan than in the United States.

Centenarians are in fact the fastest growing population group in post-industrialized countries. The rate of centenarians per 100,000 persons in the industrialized countries for 2000-2011 varies by country: 36.8 in Japan, 26.6 in Italy, 25.8 in France, 20.3 in the United Kingdom, 17.4 in Canada, 17.3 in the United States, 15.1 in Germany, and 3.8 in Russia. Japan stands out as an exception. More recent figures for Japan—with the highest centenarian rate in the world—show an increase of 46.21 per 100,000 indicating a continuing increase in both the percentage and the number of centenarians. Although most centenarians live independently until age 92, by the time they reach the century mark, half are living in nursing homes, while 15 percent are still living alone. The rest are living with someone, or in assisted living facilities. While about 85 percent are women, a community in Sardinia exists where men outlive women. Researchers indicate that centenarian tend to have extroverted personalities, and will often have many friends, strong ties to relatives and a healthy dose of self-esteem.

The Emergence of Centenarians

UC Berkeley demographer John Wilmoth, now the Director of the U.N. Population Division, estimated that the emergence of centenarians occurred around 2500 B.C., when the world population reached 100 million. This occurred at the time of the first great human civilization, the Sumerian period in Mesopotamia. The emergence of extreme longevity provides additional insight into the story of *Epic of Gilgamesh*, the first recorded story written on love, friendship and the search for immortality. The tale was conceived at a time when aging came of age. Although other demographers argue that there were no true centenarians prior to 1800, an argument mainly propounded, among others by Bernard Jeune.

Proposing that centenarians are a modern phenomenon is important not just for statistics, but also for philosophy. The great debate about the emergence of the first centenarians relates to a single issue—whether humans have changed in modern history and that we are becoming more resilient and living longer. A concept that eases the door open to exceptional longevity in the future since we are still "improving." Or the alternate interpretation that centenarians are a statistical artifact, based simply on probability. That the larger the population, the more probable that exceptional longevity will occur. As rare as centenarians are, Supercentenarians are rarer still.

Supercentenarians-breaking the 110-year barrier

We can see that centenarians do not just linger in disability and morbidity. They generally delay the onset of disease and disability. Longevity is usually a reflection of good health—until, that is, the age of 100 when both clinical and demographic evidence indicates a speedy onset of frailty and disease. At this age, centenarians come face-to-face with their lifespan. The final 10 years—from being a centenarian to becoming a supercentenarian—has the highest mortality rate of all ages. That decade, from 100 to 110, remains the most difficult to attain as a human.

Despite an incredible demographic growth among centenarians, supercentenarians remain extremely rare. Out of all centenarians, only one in two hundred will survive that extra 10 years. This presents the strongest argument for the existence of a lifespan, a barrier that restricts further longevity. Although academically we might argue for specifics of this limit—as Leonard Hayflick has proposed with a 115-year lifespan—no one can deny that a biological limit exists.

The International Database on Longevity coordinates an international collaborative effort to identify the number of validated supercentenarians. This database has identified a total of 12 supercentenarians in Sweden, 2 in Denmark, 49 in France, 78 in Japan, and 341 in the United States. Fewer than 500 supercentenarians are alive in the world at any given time. Not many studies exist that examine this unique population.

In a study looking at the health of supercentenarians and centenarians, a Japanese group led by Yasumichi Arai from Keio University School of Medicine, and his colleagues investigated 642 centenarians, including 84 supercentenarians. They found the most impressive difference occurs in terms of their score on the Mini Mental State Exam (MMSE)—a common short test to determine thinking capacity. On the MMSE supercentenarians scored lower, at 7.4 against 11.4 for centenarians. Although this indicates a decline in thinking competence, supercentenarians also had smaller variance in all of their scores. They are more homogenous then the younger centenarian group. It takes certain specific characteristics to live to 110 years of age and we are yet to find out what these are.

Specific Characteristics

The lawyer Lynn Peters Alder, by interviewing over 250 centenarians and their families, provides a compendium of centenarians' experiences. She has summarized these behaviors as eating frugally, being physical active, and not smoking or drinking excessively. They have a loving and supportive family and friends, some have religion, and lastly, they subscribe some of their longevity to their genes. This provides a positive view of centenarians with spiritual and psychological insights. Perhaps the gist of living to a hundred is a quote by Alder, who summarizes her observations "People who reach 100 are not quitters. They share a remarkable ability to renegotiate life at every turn, to accept the inevitable losses and move on." In 2010, Alex Bishop and his colleagues working with the Georgia Centenarian Study, found that happiness among these exceptionally older people—which is correlated with longevity—was determined by "congruence," which was defined by three statements– one being satisfied with life, one to have gotten what you expected out of life, and the last one: "I would not change my past life even if I could." This is the core character of supercentenarians.

"Even if I could" is an important admission. Centenarians and to a greater degree, supercentenarians, are healthier, tend to escape or delay diseases, are more cognitively competent, strong willed, and comfortable where they are. Economically, even if they are poor, they tend to feel that they have enough money. If you are getting frailer, becoming more diminished, experiencing the loss of loved-ones, friends and colleagues, and facing increasing challenges, limited options exist. None of them include reversing this trend. The best utilization of a person's energies is to accept the changes and assume that you are destined to be here (wherever "here" is). Psychologists call this a positive character-disposition and strong adaptability to the adversities of life. You are meant to be where you are. Being happy is one of the constant themes among centenarians.

Happiness

It is no surprise that happy people live longer, and happy countries have higher life expectancy. Zoologists have even documented that happy orangutans live longer. It would seem that happiness is an important commodity. Older adults often evidence a conspiracy to be happy. Not only do happy people live longer, but adults are more likely to become happier with age.

What makes us so happy? In *The Paradox of Choice: Why More Is Less*, Barry Schwartz posits that the secret for happiness is not having a great choice or achieving your goals and dreams. No. Happiness comes from accepting what you have, being happy with the choices that you made. Having more choices makes us less happy, and it does not matter what those choices are. Which is what makes Daniel Gilbert's cheerfully engaging book *Stumbling On Happiness* so good. The argument that it is not choices that make us happy, but accepting the choices we make, has generated a lot of interest. In psychology Paul Baltes's model of selection, optimization, and compensation (SOC) argues that it is essential for successful development that older adults maximize their remaining capacities and minimize their losses. We do not choose to experience losses. But we choose to accept them. In his book on baseball, *Shoeless Joe*, Canadian William Patrick Kinsella summarizes this attitude when he wrote that "Success is getting what you want; happiness is wanting what you get."

In our daily life, most of us are too concerned with success and our expression of that ambition. And we see that there is a historical precedent. This positive attitude starts earlier in life, and is not learned when you become an older adult. Accepting "bad" choices, painful loss, forgiving people, being content with what you have in terms of money and health is how you tell your body that you are happy where you are and that you are not ready to go just yet. You belong here still. Even if you could change circumstances, you would choose the same path because that is what made you. Happiness tells your body that you are still present.

Evidence for the importance of happiness also comes from the opposite condition, stress. Stress, causes damage to your body, and remains the primary killer in industrialized countries.

We learned that stress is a killer from an important study on civil servants carried out in the U.K. In this study, Michael Gideon Marmot, then with the University College London, and his colleagues designed the first of what become known as the Whitehall Studies. The original study started in 1967, following 18,000 male civil servants over ten years. The results confirmed in a second study in 1985, shows a strong association between job grade levels of civil servant employment and mortality rates from a range of causes. Men in the lowest grade (messengers, doorkeepers, etc.) had a mortality rate three times higher than that of men in the highest grade (administrators). Still, the mechanism of how stress caused disease remained elusive.

Then in 2017, a new study elucidated some of the mechanisms involved. Ahmed Tawakol with Massachusetts General Hospital and Harvard Medical School, and his colleagues, followed 293 patients for just-under four years. During this time, 22 patients developed heart disease. The researchers found that excited brain activity—in a region called the amygdala—proved to result in heart disease. This activity in the amygdala was linked to increased bone marrow activity and inflammation in the arteries, which suggest a causal path. The authors suggest that the amygdala signals to the bone marrow to produce extra white blood cells, which in turn causes the arteries to develop plaques and become inflamed, which then can cause heart attack and stroke. The brain protecting the body causes the damage. But how do we control the brain?

Geography

We have known that stress causes disease by initially looking at chemical changes in the body. Although Hans Selye wrote more than 1,700 articles promoting the idea that stress translates to physical problems, only in the last two decades have scientists been able to look at the mechanics of this connection. The first line of investigation looked at chemicals released under stress, which were known to change cell behavior and make you ill.

Recent pioneering work by Janice Kiecolt-Glaser and Ronald Glaser, professors at Ohio State University, has established the role of stress on the immune system. In an early study, they found that students' responses to hepatitis B vaccine—which mimics an infectious agent—was diminished in those with higher anxiety, higher stress and less social support. This validated an earlier finding that healing of wounds was much slower in psychologically stressed adults.

But controlling stress remains elusive. Yoga, breathing techniques, and exercise all helped, but eventually proved ineffective. The Whitehall studies concluded that a higher grade of employment protected people from a wide range of diseases. Health is mediated by our sense of control. But a much simpler study exposed how we reduce disease and illustrates how "social" human beings we truly are.

Roseto story

There is an increasing interest in the geography of aging. The Blue Zones—in Dan Buettner's analysis with the National Geographic—identified clusters across the world where people commonly live active lives past the age of 100 years. These clusters of people share common practices. Apart from not smoking, eating healthy foods, and engaging in constant moderate physical activity, the other contributing factors relate to family and social engagement. Scientists have seen the identification of these Blue Zones (and other emerging clusters) as an opportunity to understand their secret, but that magic ingredient has continued to elude discovery. Buettner ascribes this longevity to a variety of factors—diet, activity and community identification. But although all these "longevity" factors are also shared with their children, we do not see their children experiencing the same level of longevity advantage as their parents. One factor that separates the older generation from the new one is the identification with a "tribe." There is some corroborating evidence for this assertion in a little known study in the United States.

Between 1955 and 1965, in Roseto, an Italian-American community in Pennsylvania, a local physician, Stewart Wolf, and later sociologist John Bruhn, observed that the locals seemed immune from heart disease—the main killer among older adults. Rosetans contradict medical knowledge to this day because their diet and risk behaviors should have resulted in diminished health status. They smoked old-style Italian very strong stogie cigars, fried food in animal fat (lard), and ate cholesterol-rich salami and cheeses. Both genders drank copious amounts of wine in preference to soft drinks or milk. In addition, Rosetan men worked in slate quarries that were not only toxic but also environmentally dangerous. Socially, the neighboring English and Welsh ethnic communities shunned them, and they themselves shunned others. But in contrast to such adverse conditions, the community reported no crime and few people registered to receive social assistance. More importantly, there was very little ostentatious inequity. Everyone lived modestly as one large family as they did before they emigrated from the same village of Roseto south of Rome. A strange observation was that for more than two decades they had very low rates of heart disease. But then these differences disappeared because of one change.

In the 1980s, with increasing acculturation, Roseto's health benefits began to erode. New residents started coming into the community, older residents died or moved away, and over a period of a decade the composition of the community changed. With this loss of community came diseases. The lesson Roseto teaches us more than half a century later, is that geography by itself is not enough. It is identifying a place with its people, culture and family–which seems to have protective function. A sense of family grounded in a particular geography protects the body from disease, and might promote extreme longevity. Such insight might explain the clustering of centenarians. This is what we see throughout the Blue Zones.

Geography is important because it reflects that sense of family, where family "has your back." You do not need to be on high alert all the time. Your stress level is low, confirming the Whitehall studies results. Your brain relaxes knowing that a whole community supports you. But is there other activity that relaxes the brain enough, to protect itself, to stop sending dangerous messages to the body?

Sex

Pragmatically we know that sex, and the activity surrounding sex, decreases stress but does it also increase longevity? Howard Friedman and Leslie Martin in the *Longevity Project* analyzed the results from a longitudinal study and provided a first glimpse into female orgasms and longevity. The study, which was begun by Lewis Terman of Stanford University in 1921 on 1,548 children with high intelligence born around 1910, was continued after his death in 1958. Now with the participants in their nineties, the study morphed into a gerontological study. One of the interesting and pertinent findings was that women who had a higher frequency of orgasm tended to live longer than their less-fulfilled women in the study.

No data on men was collected from this study. But a separate study in in the town of Caerphilly in South Wales, England, provided evidence for males. George Davey Smith with the Department of Social Medicine, University of Bristol, and his colleagues interviewed nearly 1,000 men in six small villages about their sexual activity frequency, then followed up on their death records ten years later. The authors determined that men who had two or more orgasms a week had died at a rate half that of the men who had orgasms less than once a month. And importantly, a dose effect emerged, where the more times these men had orgasms the longer they lived. These observations have been replicated in Sweden and in the USA for both males and females.

For centenarians, although there is anecdotal evidence that sexual activity is "rampant," surveys show that at that age, there is a general lack of interest in sex. Although exceptions exist, the evidence shows that centenarians have greater satisfaction with life and with social and family relations than do younger individuals. Magazine reports tend to highlight the exceptions, but in general it seems that the frequency of sex diminishes with age, especially for women whose partner has died. As most centenarians are women, perhaps the reality is less sexy to report. Perhaps there are many ways to tell the body that it is not quite finished yet. But we like the stories of sex among centenarians because it proves to us that there is still vigor with extreme longevity, we still have hope to dream that we can have both vigor and longevity.

Exceptional

We want to retain our youth for longer periods of our lives. But we should heed the lesson of Tithonus, a mythological Trojan king whose lover's father–the god Zeus–granted him immortality but not eternal youth. He eventually became so wrinkled and incapacitated that his lover turned him into a cicada—eternally living, but begging for death. What we seek is not just longevity but vigor, and a lot of older adults are finding it and holding on to it.

Louis Armstrong was 66-years-and-10-months-old when his career peaked with "What A Wonderful World" and "Cabaret" in 1968. Armstrong joins many who continued to be especially productive into older age. Numerous examples exist of artists, actors, writers and academicians who continue to produce great work at older age. A half-century ago, Harvey Lehman showed that our most creative period is between ages 33-36. But the formula is not prescriptive, and exceptions are common. When it comes to health and longevity, we all want to be the exception. It is not that we just want to live longer, it is that we want to live longer, healthier and more productively.

More and more older adults are breaking conventional expectations about physical barriers. In 2006, Maria del Carmen Bousada Lara gave birth to twin boys in Barcelona, Spain. Nothing seems remarkable about that except Lara was within a week of her 67th birthday. Although older adults are breaking records across the board, 2002 was a banner year. Tamae Watanabe reached the summit of Mt Everest at the age of 63. Jenny Wood-Allen completed the London Marathon at 90-years-old. James Talbot Guyer parachuted off the 148-meter high Perrine Bridge near Twin Falls, Idaho at age 74 years. More recently, Robert McKeague, age 80, completed the 2005 Ford Ironman World Championship. Two years later, Linda Ashmore swam the English Channel at age 60. After that, Bahadur Sherchan reached the highest point on Earth—summiting Mount Everest at the age of 76. And more recently, in 2016, a Frenchman Robert Marchand, who previously broke cycling record in over-100s category, made history by cycling more than 14 miles in an hour at the age of 105. It seems that a lot more older adults are reaching older age while they are still healthy and active. This secret helps explain the increase in the number of centenarians.

James W. Vaupel & Bernard Jeune with the Max Planck Institute have written extensively on centenarian statistics. They observe that an increase in the number of centenarians indicates that survival chances of getting there have improved. This might seem simplistic—that the growth in centenarians is largely attributable to an increase in the probability of an octogenarian becoming a centenarian—but it holds an answer to extreme longevity. As life expectancy increases from 20 to 80, the chance of surviving from birth to age 50 grows about 5-fold and the chance of surviving from 50 to 80 increases roughly 15 fold. Remarkable as these changes are, they are dwarfed by the 5,000-fold multiplication of the chance of surviving from 80 to 100.

There is both a safer environment in terms of public health, and also enhanced resilience among individuals.

Being rich helps. Although not all centenarians are rich, rich people are more likely to survive to older age then poor people. The secret with money is not being rich but having enough, an issue that can be very subjective. Although researchers found that 67 percent of 100-year-olds had income below the poverty line, 95 percent indicated to the researchers that they had enough money to meet their needs, and 76 percent of these poor centenarians even reported they had "enough to buy extras." It is very much a subjective evaluation.

Escapers and Delayers

Centenarians and to a greater extent, supercentenarians, are truly unique individuals. When Thomas Perl and his colleagues looked at whether these individuals were just more resilient then the rest of the human population they found a mixture of conditions, especially for centenarians. But for supercentenarians they found very distinct conditions. Perl and his colleagues examined 424 centenarians (aged 97-119 years), looking at the frequency of diagnoses of hypertension, heart disease, diabetes, stroke, non-skin cancer, skin cancer, osteoporosis, thyroid condition, Parkinson's disease, chronic obstructive pulmonary disease and cataracts. They excluded cognitive impairment, which might have held some interesting clues. But even without this, Perl and his colleagues found some interesting evidence. By distinguishing individuals on their history, they came up with three distinct categories:

- Survivors, those who had a diagnosis of an illness prior to the age of 80.

- Delayers, individuals who delayed the onset of an illness until at least the age of 80
- Escapers, individuals who attained their 100th year of life without the diagnosis of common age-associated illnesses.

Most female centenarians were survivors and delayers, with only 1 in 7 being escapers. Women have more illnesses from which they survive, and men tend to die more easily from their illnesses. For centenarian men, more than a third were escapers and nearly half were delayers. Like the general population, centenarian men are more likely to die then women. But even more interesting is what happens to supercentenarians. By the time that they reach 110, more than half are escapers, while a quarter are delayers. The extreme of longevity is not populated by people who have overcome diseases, but by people who have escaped disease. This probability is also seen in the progression to extreme old age.

Supercentenarians have evaded or delayed disease. Despite such impressive resilience, it is wise not to paint them as caricatures in a marvel comic. Without exception, after their 110th birthdays all supercentenarians become frail and eventually spend their last years confined to wheelchairs, virtually blind, very hard of hearing and invariably institutionalized. A handful makes it past 115, most extremely frail. But up to the final shutdown of the body, there an undeniable resilience remains apparent. Similarly, an undeniable barrier exists that ends in death proceeded by extreme frailty. It might be possible that by looking at a population we can surmise patterns that identify way we eventually have to die.

Patterns

Centenarians and supercentenarians are showing us that the human body can deflect diseases for a very long period of time, but once the barrier has been penetrated, the decline is certain and fast. In a convergence of thought we come back to the Gompertz-Makeham curve–that mortality is a combination of constant threat from the environment (Makeham) and the increasing risk of death as we get older (Gompertz). The dominant scientists in this field, the husband and wife team of Leonid Gavrilov and Natalia Gavrilova, have focused on the problem of whether the vulnerability to diseases—as predicted by the Gompertz curve—eventually kills centenarians rather than environmental factors. Once resilience is breached, the constant presence of diseases takes over—the Makeham constant.

In agreement with demographers, Gavrilov and Gavrilova argue that the overall decline of mortality during the last century has been due to better public health–a reduction in the Makeham curve, making it more likely that octogenarians become nonagenarians and then centenarians. But the curve is not accurate. At very young, and very old ages, the curve does not accurately reflect death rates, which are higher for newborns and lower for centenarians. This observation has generated numerous speculations.

All of these questions contributed to the 1980 Larry Heligman and John Hurlstone Pollard model, which explains early infant death and early adult mortality, but does not explain mortality at later ages very well. The importance of this slight advantage at very old age is that it provides scientists with the possibility that there are unique conditions at this stage in life. Others have tried to adjust older-age death rates–in particular, William Perks, Robert Beard and Väinö Kannisto, among many others. Although they have improved upon the formula—producing a curve that accounts for the slowing of death for the oldest old—they propose no explanation other than "greater variance among this group." Unlike the Heligman-Pollard model, which defines the three behavioral and clinical components that produce their estimate, the Perks-Beard-Kannisto model for older age has very little explanation for the decline in mortality in extreme old age. These are all technical issues. The significance of these explorations indicates that we do not have a clue what is happening at much later age, and we cannot even find a model that expresses this advantage. These scientists are basically saying that even within this group of centenarians, some people are going to live much longer than others. But this is a circular argument and does not explain why.

Familial Connection

Without making any assumptions of whether this is due to genetics or the environment—since we already have seen how muddled that false dichotomy is—we observe that daughters of centenarians live 10 years longer on average. This indicates that long-lived people are fundamentally different from other people in the sense that their children also live significantly longer lives. Although it would be logical to assume a genetic link, and there must be, the relationship, as we have seen, is likely to be less direct. By looking at everyone within a population, it seems that they are varied, and they are. But if we identify them earlier on, we can see that while the rest of the population falls away, the resilient few remain. We know who these unique, resilient people are. The point of separation—according to demography but as yet not biology—is at about age 85 for mothers. At this age, close to life expectancy, death becomes much more selective. You can exercise, eat well, keep your weight down, live healthily, refrain from smoking, drink alcohol in measured amounts, take holidays and take control of life. That will get you to the precipice, a life expectancy of around 85 years of age. Anything beyond is unknown. The importance of the Gompertz-Makeham-Perks equation is that it tells us that once we reach this age, the rate of death slows down. Although many conjectures exist, there remains no answer to why we observe this in extreme old age.

One of the earliest studies in the United States that examined this idea took place more than a hundred years ago, in 1918. A famous scientist was looking at birth and death records to identify familial patterns in extreme longevity of centenarians. Although earlier studies had looked at centenarians—in Chinese families in the 14th-19th century and Swedish families between 1500-1829—and none other than Alexander Graham Bell conducted the one in the USA. Famous for inventing the telephone (among other things), he was also one of the first to undertake a systematic study of centenarians.

Bell based his work on an earlier study by Reuben Walworth (1864) using some meticulously detailed 8,797 records of descendants of William Hyde who died in 1681. This extended family were early settlers of Norwich, Connecticut. While most of the descendants died before age 40—a testament to the hazardous environmental conditions which prevailed at the time—a small minority survived till very old age. Overall, Bell found females dying at higher proportions before 40 years of age—likely due to the dangers of childbirth—after which women began gaining an increasing survival advantage. Bell identified that the longevity of parents (more so for fathers) related to the longevity of their children. Interestingly he found that longer lived parents had more children, while fathers who married younger lived longer.   Bell's very perceptive in observations included that "…long-lived people, though few in number, may profoundly affect the composition of the whole population born in the next generation." (p.52). Later he concluded that "…the very fact of their surviving to old age proved themselves to be resistant to disease…Here we have evidence of a natural process at work among human beings, tending to improve the vigor and vitality of succeeding generations." (p.53).

This familial relationship holds true today as well. Centenarians comprise a homogenous group—with few exceptions. They are mainly women, with 7 out of ten of all centenarians. Physically, few are obese especially men, and they rarely have a substantial smoking history–although around one in five smoked in the past. Jeane Louise Calment smoked until she was 117, and she only stopped because she became blind and had difficulty lighting up. But she smoked only two to three cigarettes a day.   One in seven lucky centenarians experience no significant changes in their cognition. Many centenarian women have a history of bearing children after the age of 35 years. At least half of centenarians have first-degree relatives and/or grandparents who also achieve very old age, and many have exceptionally old siblings.   Male siblings of centenarians have a 17 times greater chance than other men born around the same time of reaching age 100 years. While female siblings of centenarians have an 8½ greater chance than other females of attaining age 100. Such familial influence cannot be due to chance and must be due to factors that members of these families have in common. Whether these factors are innate or external is still muddled, but genetic variation plays a very strong role in exceptional longevity. But does not determine it, it promotes longevity.

We have known, since Bell's observations at the turn of the 20th century, that biological relatives of centenarians have substantial survival advantages compared to others. By looking at parents, spouses, siblings and siblings-in-law of centenarians—because they have known similarities in their environment, upbringing and social class—demographers can examine the genetic influence on longevity. The findings from such studies indicate that for males, having a centenarian brother is associated with longer life than having a centenarian sister. For fathers, having a centenarian son is associated with increased longevity than having a centenarian daughter. Sex of centenarians is important in influencing the longevity of siblings but not for siblings-in-law. Only women benefit from having centenarian spouse. Overall, these studies emphasize a genetic component as promoting rather than determining longevity, and that such familial factors in human longevity are likely to be sex-specific. This means that if there are genetic markers they are likely to be on the sex chromosome. Females are ten times more likely than men to become centenarians. But there are exceptions, which is how the study of Blue Zones started when Michel Poulain validated a group of men in Sardinia that lived longer than women. The fact that this area in Sardinia was mountainous seems to have some advantage. In South Korea, the physician Sang Chul Park observed that centenarian men are more common in mountainous areas, compared to centenarian women who cluster by the seashore or in flat areas. It is not simply a gene here and there. The surprise is that recent studies have continued to erode the genetic card in longevity.

Real Life Stories of Genetic Influence

Genes only promote, but do not determine longevity, and we do not know how. One contrary argument is that long-lived individuals do not have genes that cause disease. Such mechanistic interpretations become quickly discounted when scrutinized. Marian Beekman and her colleagues from Leiden University found genes known for increasing the risk of coronary artery disease, cancer, and type 2 diabetes, among long-lived individuals from long-lived families as well as in young controls from regular families. Longevity in this study population is not compromised by the cumulative effect of genes that increase the risk for common disease. The decisive critique of a genetic control of longevity, however—whether it is one gene or many—comes from the 2016 study by Rong Chen, Stephen Friend and Eric Schadt from the Icahn School of Medicine and their colleagues who found that even Mendelian genetic diseases are not solely caused by genetics (reported in chapter 2).

Two possible interpretations account for this outcome: that the Mendelian diseases identified were in fact incorrectly defined and there might be other genes involved (more than two alleles). Secondly, that these individuals are resilient to the disease. That there are other factors— including other genes, epigenetic influence and other biological mechanisms—that determine whether the disease emerges. One of the surprising components, showing great promise in explaining diseases, is the micro-organisms that live with us. This microbiota—the group of micro-organisms lives with us–includes bacteria, viruses and archaea (single cell organisms with no cell nucleus). We have seen how the microbiota of humans not only act as organs in our bodies by influencing our chemical signals and conditions, but an exchange of genetic material also occurs. We have recently discovered that centenarians and supercentenarians have different bacteria then younger populations.

Bacteria

In northern Italy, researchers studied the gut bacteria of centenarians. They found that the microbiota of centenarians is significantly less diverse than that of elderly (60–80 years old) and young adults (20–40 years old), and that they had more bad bacteria such as bacilli. When the gut bacteria of centenarians were compared to their children's (average age 67.5 years) no similarity was found, indicating that the change was due to age and not familial factors. Although the composition of the microbiome differs across countries (e.g. China), a general pattern was discovered. Among older adults there is decreasing diversity in types of bacteria and an increase in certain types of bacteria was found.

In 2016, Elena Biagi, and her colleagues with the University of Bologna, looked at the stomach bacteria of semi-supercentenarians—those 105 years and older—and found a microbial system enriched in beneficial health-promoting bacteria. The composition was different between these semi-supercentenarians and younger (99-104 years old) individuals. Could gut bacteria be related to when you were born rather than age? Were these healthy bacteria already present at a younger age, which might explain why these individuals survived to such extreme age? Or alternatively did these individuals re-acquire the bacteria as they got much older (e.g., through a less varied diet). The likely answer, as we have explored through this book, is all three possibilities, with an additional twist. Bacteria also reside everywhere on the body and in large numbers in the lungs, mouth, skin and sex organs. Recent evidence suggests that the age-related changes in gut and lung microbiota may also influence health in other parts of the body–not just the stomach. Of particular interest is the finding that poor oral hygiene results in oral bacteria invading the heart as well as the brain.

Elena Biagi's work with 24 semi-supercentenarians— 105 years and older—and 15 centenarians, reported this "invasion" of bacteria from other parts of the body. But rather than seeing this as an invasion, in our study of immortality, a better perspective might interpret it as communication. Extremely long-living people seem to experience an increase in several health-promoting bacteria— in particular, from the bacteria families *Christensenellaceae*, *Akkermansia* and *Bifidobacterium*—well-known health- associated bacteria families that help the immune system, protect against inflammation, and promote a healthy metabolic balance. It is likely that for long-lived individuals, a cohort effect exists. When (and perhaps where) you are born determines the bacteria in your body. That behavior and diet determines the type and level of bacteria. With increasing age this bacteria changes, influenced by bacteria from other parts of the body. Whether these bacteria changes promote or demote health is determined by still-unknown factors. It could be that beneficial microbiota is promoted earlier in development, and that some conditions at birth promote a healthier environment than others.

Seasonality

A clue, that resilience to disease might be a long-term factor, emerges from the conditions at birth. The German scientist Gabriele Doblhammer with the University of Rostock and his colleagues with the Max Planck Institute, have been looking at how seasons determine longevity. Doblhammer reported that individuals born in September to February (dipping slightly in November) live longer than individuals born in any other month. Leonid Gavrilov and Natalia Gavrilova corroborated these results, finding the same consistent pattern. People born in September–November are more likely to survive to 100 years of age than individuals born in March.

Several explanations exist for season-of birth effects on longevity, pointing to the effects of early-life conditions that determine later-life outcomes. Initial environmental factors can determine this. For example, there is a reduction in initial exposure to bacteria and viruses that have seasonal cycles (e.g. influenza virus peaks from November to March), availability of food (such seasonal availability was more evident in the past), temperature and sun exposure. Theoretically, some emerging explanations go beyond environmental factors. The role of epigenetics, as a way of marrying the environment with the biology, is a prime contender since epigenetic influences can have long lasting effects. As we have seen in previous chapters, the environment poses a constant threat (Makeham), and reduced resilience (Gompertz) that comes with older ages. Seasonally effects can influence both types of factors.

Obviously, reducing exposure to infectious disease and other sources of inflammation in children results in a decline in old-age mortality. The idea of a 'cohort morbidity phenotype'—identified among animals but applicable to humans as well—suggests that early-life trauma causes inflammation, that progress to chronic long-terms diseases in middle age. These traumas can be caused by adverse environmental conditions, food deprivation, or other external events. Such traumas can also be seasonal. In such cases, there will be cohort effects in a group born around the same time—either positive or negative.

Mismatch Hypothesis

The concept that our longevity—and therefore our health—is determined by events that happens outside of our control and before we are born is antithetic to the modern day anti-aging movement. Initially proposed by James Neel at the University of Michigan in 1962, it is incorrectly referred to as the "thrifty gene" hypothesis, because sometimes people are pre-disposed to store fat more than others, especially within deprived communities. This happens because if a fetus experiences deprived nutrition, the epigenes become tuned to expect a meager supply of nutrients—an inappropriate adaptation for later nutritional excess. Lack of nutrition in fetal development or periodic famines in the past while still in uterus, switch on epigenetic activity that maximizes metabolic efficiency—by storing nutrients in fat and promote food-access behaviors. The mismatch between fetal conditions and outside environmental conditions causes problems for biology. This "Mismatch Theory" is not without its eugenic undertones. We can easily classify poor people's risk behaviors as a "thrifty gene" syndrome. But the reality is very different from this criticism.

The evidence comes from two very different geographical regions–the Netherlands and Russia. During the Dutch Hunger Winter, which lasted six months during 1944-1945, Germans blockaded the western Netherlands. At one point the population relied on less than a third of their nutritional requirements. Some were reduced to eating grass and tulip bulbs. More than 20,000 people died. But the fact that all of the community suffered just one specific period of malnutrition was unlike the siege of Leningrad (the modern-day St. Petersburg) that lasted 872 days. It killed over two million people, including 800,000 civilians. It began on September 8, 1941 when German and Finnish troops encircled the city and cut it off from supplies. A dystopian story emerged as the unforgiving Russian winter depleted water supplies and fuel and residents, with only half of the allowance provided to their Dutch counterparts, ate anything they could to survive. One obvious impact was on pregnant women and the low birth weights of children born just after the blockade. Comparing the babies born after the siege of Leningrad with babies exposed to the Dutch Hunger Winter proved perplexing at first. Whereas both babies born after the blockade were born small, there was a major difference in the long-term consequences, which has subsequently been replicated. The results were perplexing but insightful for us in our exploration of immortality.

Whereas the babies born after the Dutch Hunger Winter resumed a normal diet, the babies born after the Siege of Leningrad experienced continuing food shortages. These post-blockade conditions had dramatic effects on the babies but not the way we would expect. For the Leningrad children, being exposed to famine in utero, although they were born small, they did not exhibit higher rates of either obesity or cardio vascular disease later on as adults even though they still experienced food shortage as they were growing up. However, for the Dutch newborns that faced a much richer nutritional environment than the one experienced in uterus, as adults they experienced long lasting physical and mental health issues. We still see these effects today with death rates from heart disease being five times higher among men who were thin at birth but became overweight by age eleven.

If a mother was well-fed around the time of conception and malnourished only for the last few months of the pregnancy, her baby was likely to be born small. But if the mother suffered malnutrition only for the first three months of the pregnancy but then resumed a normal diet—after the blockade ended—the baby was born normal size. The fetus "caught up" in body weight. Subsequent long-term studies have also shown that not just weight was affected, but also longevity and mental health. Despite them having caught-up, long-term negative consequences resulted. The study about the Dutch Hunger Winter was published in 1976, suggesting that maternal malnutrition during gestation may permanently affect adult health without affecting the size of the baby at birth. It implied that the quick adaptations that enable the fetus to continue to grow might nevertheless have adverse consequences in later life.

The only available interpretation was that it was not simply a matter of nutritional deficit but the timing of such shocks. How does the fetus know what environment is waiting outside? And why are there such negative consequences when it gets it wrong? At the time in the late 1970s, no explanation materialized for these observations. Then came a unique concept of disease.

Barker Hypothesis

These observations set the foundation for the early 1980s studies by David Barker with the British Medical Research Council Environmental Epidemiology Unit (now the Lifecourse Epidemiology Unit). Barker, using British epidemiological data, noted that although overall rates of cardiovascular disease increase with rising national prosperity, the poorest suffer the highest rates of disease. Over a series of studies Barker and others proposed that an adverse fetal environment followed by plentiful food in adulthood might be a recipe for adult chronic disease, a claim referred to as the "Barker Hypothesis" or "fetal programming hypothesis." The proposition that the environment of the fetus and infant—controlled by the mother's nutrition and the baby's exposure to infection after birth determines diseases in later life was at the time seen as preposterous and laughable. Undeterred, Barker believed that public health was failing. He believed that we could eradicate most diseases by protecting the nutrition of young women. The Barker Hypothesis is re-emerging as an important milestone in understanding health and therefore longevity.

If nutritional variance during fetal growth has long-term consequences, then such variance can also be created not only by famines as a result of blockades and natural disasters–and also as a result of natural seasonal and historic variations in food supply. It could be that the year of birth, which acts as a proxy for the food abundance or dearth, could similarly determine not only birth weight but also long term physical and mental development, including longevity.

Seasonal Death

Actuaries—statisticians that look at data in order to calculate insurance risks and premiums—were the first to notice that year of birth was a powerful predictor of disease. The year of birth predicts exposure and susceptibility to disease and risk behaviors. In some instances, year of birth is more important than age and the year of observation. Year of birth is a better predictor of dying from stroke than age. There is also a generational effect. Because these changes modify which genes are switched on and off, the changes jump to subsequent generations. For example, a Norwegian study reported that stillbirth rates are more closely linked to the mother's own year of birth than the year of the stillbirth itself.

The success of statisticians in predicting individual lifespan—age at death—developed into the "cohort morbidity phenotype." People born during a certain period of time, share (ill) health characteristics. The husband and wife team of Leonid Gavrilov and Natalia Gavrilova have written extensively about this process of early influence and the effect of high initial damage load on longevity. The conditions in the womb and the process of birth itself are important in determining lifelong health. Year of birth can be a useful proxy for both early-life conditions and lifetime effects, so much so that the British statisticians Stephen Richards, John Kirby and Iain Currie continue to show that mortality patterns can be made to fit better by using year of birth rather than age. Although period effects exist as well—related to the culture at a specific time such as the prevalence of smoking, which was higher than today— period effects do not eliminate all the cohort effects.

A twist in this story occurred when in the late 1970s, Hans Eysenck and David Nias began publishing work showing a correlation between the year and date of birth and a series of characteristics that they then correlated to marriage, illness, suicide, physical appearance, earthquakes and career choice. These works followed from the earlier and much maligned work of the Parisian Michel Gauquelin (1928-1991) and his Swiss-born wife Francoise (1929-2007). The Gauquelins had earlier proposed that planetary positions correlate with the personality of 17,000 eminent professionals. Michel Gauquelin, a statistical psychologist found that eminent people tended to be born in seasons where a specific planet's diurnal position was closer or farther from earth. Specifically, the Gauquelins found that Mars was significant for physicians, military leaders and sports champions, Jupiter for actors, and Saturn for scientists. Mars and Saturn also showed a deficit for painters. By 1978 these observations were later analyzed by Tom Shanks and the computer of Neil Michelsen's Astro

Computing Service now in New Hampshire, USA. The results were positive but there remained some technical issues with the interpretation of results—mainly the effect of large samples causing false negatives (known as type 2 error), how traits are defined for correlation, and the cut-off point for deciding on the diurnal cycle of the planets, among other methodological issues. Although statistical significance does not tell us how strong these effects were, the fact that there was an effect proved providential in promoting early influences. Specifically, they speculated that the unborn child might have a particular planetary sensitivity.

This would not have been news except that Hans Jurgen Eysenck started replicating their findings in the 1970s. As a professor of psychology at the Institute of Psychiatry in London, Eysenck was arguably the most influential psychologist of his time. His unswerving allegiance to the scientific method meant that those that had the temerity to cross swords with him had to do it on the battlefield of science. Eysenck always won. Eysenck's contributions to astrological research were his insistence that there was an effect to be explained, and although he could not explain the outcome his insistence that matters needed to be resolved by appropriate experiments meant that he refused to be satisfied with dismissive explanations. To this day, we have no explanation for these statistically significant outcomes.

Recent studies continue exposing the effect of moon phase on fertility, sleep patterns, recovery from operations, heart rate and blood pressure. While solar storms have been linked to rheumatoid arthritis. As recently as 2015 Nick Tatonetti, with Columbia University Medical Center continues the tradition, linking month of birth to the prevalence of 55 distinct diseases. Overall, the study indicated people born in May had the lowest disease risk, and those born in October the highest.

These studies all point in one direction. That our bodies and our minds are designed to respond to the environment and that this preparation starts at inception. And we share this world together with our partners in life— our resident bacteria, viruses, fungi and protozoa—our own symbionts.

The biology of immortality needs to address this reality in order to explain longevity. Seeing that long life reflects good health suggests that longevity might be simply be the result of not dying, not being prone to killer diseases, or delaying killer diseases. We either escape or delay diseases by being resilient to them. Our environment in the womb, as well as while we are growing in childhood and early adult life have predisposed us to live healthier and therefore longer. But then how we behave, or a changing environment, might negate this biological advantage.

As the mismatch theory suggests, we might be designed for a sparing nutritional environment, but once we are born we face the opposite environment, a rich nutritional environment, then our efficient biology overcompensates. We end up storing too much energy through fat, and we know only too well how that story unfolds in later life. Alternatively, we might experience a very rich nutritional environment in the womb and our biology adjusts to slow down the storage of fat (as an example)–only to face a diminished nutritional environment once we are born. This may result in a stunted and comprised growth. Once we are conceived, our biology is continually modifying us to survive. As we continue to learn throughout our exploration in this book, longevity is a part of this package. It does not seem to be separate from resilience to diseases.

Biological life is a balance between what was expected and what we experience. For example, Dutch Hendrikje van Andel Schipper, was born prematurely, with a weight of only three pounds. But she lived to enjoy her 115th birthday. Because she was deprived in the fetus, and then experienced great scarcity—as a result of the German occupation during the Second World War, her fetal condition and her outside world matched. She survived by selling her jewelry to buy food. Her survival is also a testament to the "grandmother effect," since as a frail premature baby she was tended by her grandmother during the first month of her frail life, enabling her to survive and then thrive. Being born prematurely and then experiencing great deprivation may explain how she lived in harmony with the environment. Although when it came to examining this capacity for longevity, an international team lead by Henne Holstege from the VU University Medical Center in Amsterdam, identified that stem cells were protecting her white blood cell telomeres. Many newspapers and magazines took this as a binary answer and plastered their front page with "Stem Cells Cure Aging." What they do not report is that Schipper also survived a mastectomy from breast cancer and her autopsy found a malignant tumor "the size of a small fist" in her stomach. There are no binary answers but a balance. This balance goes back in history as well as crossing from the individual to the environment.

Conclusion of lessons from centenarians

It could be that having lived so long, centenarians have developed immunity. They gained immune capital–hat after a certain adult age, the older they live the more resilient they become. It seems, therefore, that centenarians are still gaining an advantage. Early influences, as proposed by the Barker Hypothesis determine health and longevity.

Environmental stability ensures that centenarians are biological programmed correctly in the womb to meet the environment that they live in. It could also be seasonal. They might have been exposed to the right types of bacteria growing up, or that their genes responded appropriately and adequately to environmental stressors. We cannot determine the exact mechanism for their advantage but we know that all these factors contribute to longevity. The low hanging fruit is that it reflects genes, diet and exercise. But this is not a comprehensive story. People who diet, exercise and have familial longevity are more likely to die before their 100th birthday than to celebrate it. We are still discussing what makes centenarians so special—especially since the children and grandchildren of those in the Blue Zone are themselves not reaching the same age as their parents.

It could also be, especially for supercentenarians, that they might be a product of our time. Could it be that these long-lived individuals are truly so exceptional that they emerged at a special time in our history and might disappear altogether in the future? This might not be such a strange prediction; especially if we appreciate that centenarians might not always have been part of our populations.

The lessons from life expose a much broader interplay than our current focus on genetics, biology or pharmacology allows. Real world observations point to the importance of history and the environment. We can talk about culture, spirituality and a sense of belonging, but that is premature. We need science to catch up with such nuanced thinking. Just appreciating the importance of our developmental history and the relationship that our biology has with our micro-organisms—our symbionts—and the environment is sufficiently radical by itself. Gerontology has broadened the exploration of longevity by addressing our historical relationship with environmental stressors (i.e. seasonal variation and food availability) and symbionts (bacteria, viruses, fungi and protozoa.)

Our analyses of real life lessons broaden our search for the mechanism of extreme longevity and highlight the need to be in tune with our immediate environment. Longevity reflects a global assessment of health throughout our lives. There cannot be a longevity gene or longevity biology, there are only healthy genes and a healthy biology. What makes them healthy is that they are in concert with the environment. Nothing is determined everything is negotiated with our environment. The only place that determinism exists, that simplistic binary idea of cause and effect, is in our psychology. In the real world, no panacea, no single change exists that can dramatically change the course of longevity.

Although many activities and behaviors contribute to longevity, these are only useful up to a point. With extreme longevity you will need to survive all of these different sequential stages. Mark Edmundson the University of Virginia professor of literature could have been referring to centenarians when he said that "In later life most good things happen very slowly; only bad things tend to happen fast." There are observable differences between centenarians and their younger cohorts. Most of the science has focused on diet, exercise and social context. We are now examining broader influences such as mismatch theory, bacteria, early environmental experiences, and a sense of belonging. How bacteria colonize us while in the womb and then develop with us as we grow older is a story that remains to be told. Differences between the bacteria in the gut of centenarians compared to supercentenarians expose how little we still know. As a result of this complexity, our current approach to dissect and look at specific events is not tenable. In order to understand the mechanism, we have to stand back and look at the choreography. Behind these physical observations lies something grander. Even if we detail the complexity of our biology; our genes, chemistry, biology, microbiota, social relations, psychology and spirituality, if we do not appreciate their cohesion we will lose the ability to understand longevity. We can examine the dance, but without the music we will not understand why they are dancing. We will never understand longevity nor our own ambition for immortality.

———————————∞———————————

Chapter 6

Death Fear

Whether it is the anarchy of disordered biochemistry or the direct result of its opposite—a carefully orchestrated genetic ride to death—we die of old age because we have been worn and torn and programmed to cave in. The very old do not succumb to disease—they implode their way into eternity. (p.83)

— Sherwin Nuland (1995) *How We Die Vintage.*

Death by old age was abolished in United States in 1951 when a federal Public Health Conference on Records and Statistics standardized causes of death throughout the nation omitted, by design, death by old age. With 130 competing diagnostic alternatives, age as a cause of death is no longer viable. When physicians intuitively know that death was because of old age they select "failure to thrive" as one of the 130 options available. This construct includes being physically frail, malnourished, depressed or cognitively impaired. Although eliminating old age as a cause of death promotes more specificity about conditions of death—conditions and not causes since brain death is the cause of death— theoretically it is possible to die of old age, but there are many ways to die other than old age

In truth, only one real cause of death exists—oxygen starvation to the brain. The cause of death listed on death certificates is really the cause "of" the cause, as simple as this might seem. Requirement to list a cause other than "old age" is based on the Sixth Revision of the International Lists of Diseases and Causes of Death. This revision, published in in 1948, was developed to generate data on a potentially remediable condition—death. Death can be cured. This explains why many medical euphemisms for death are expressions of failure: could not save him, lost him, expired, gone, among many others. Death has, in many senses, become a medical failure and no longer forms part of the natural cycle of life.

An estimated 100 billion people have died since humans emerged on earth. As a result, by now we should know something about dying. In 19th-century Europe there was much fear about death–not surprisingly since people were still being mistakenly buried alive. From ancient history, cadavers were laid out in "hospitals for the dead" while attendants awaited signs of "decomposition, disintegration, and separation," the Catholic definition of death. This indeterminable period is also ritualized in the Jewish (Shemira) where the soul is said to remain attached to the body for three to seven days after death. This is unlike

Muslim burial rites where the body is buried quickly after death. All religions practice the ritual of viewing the body of the deceased—with such euphemisms as Funeral Visitation, Calling Hours, Reviewal, or a Wake—making sure that the person we are about to bury is truly dead. But how difficult is it to make such a mistake?

Lyall Watson in his classic book *The Romeo Error: A Matter of Life and Death* talks about such errors–horrific errors where people are unintentionally buried alive only to be found when the tomb was exhumed or rarely, when they succeeded in escaping. After more than 350,000 years of burying homo sapiens, we should have learned how to identify death so that we do not make such grave mistakes. What remains surprisingly difficult to this day is how to define a sharp line between living and dead.

The 1981 USA Uniform Determination of Death Act (UDDA), states that patients may be pronounced legally dead either when they meet the traditional criteria for death—the cessation of breathing and the absence of a heartbeat—or when they are diagnosed as brain dead. Brain dead can refer to just the cortical brain—the top layer of the brain—showing no signs of activity, or it might also include cessation of activity in the brain stem—which control other involuntary bodily functions like breathing and digestion. Surprisingly, UDDA was never codified into law, and as a result, its application varies from hospital to hospital. Although this protocol was reviewed and improved in 1997 by the U.S. Institute of Medicine, the definition has remained structurally the same. Such a definition is a compromise between the clinical/legal and the scientific. Unfortunately, what we have today is a legal definition, not a scientific one. And such a clear-cut definition of death is legally necessary—if not altogether scientifically accurate—

for a number of conditions, one of which is organ transplantation.

Legality of Death

No discussion of brain death can take place without a companion discussion of organ transplantation. Transplanting organs need to be alive to be viable. The ideal situation for transplantation would be to have a dead body with live organs. The only way to get that is to keep the body alive while the brain is classified as dead. In cases of homicides, keeping the body alive until harvesting their organs makes a complicated legal argument—who brought about the donor's death?

In 1968—a year after the South African surgeon Christiaan N. Barnard performed the world's first human heart transplant—Stanford University surgeon Norman Shumway performed the first USA heart transplant from a brain-dead donor. These were nearly identical surgical procedures, except whereas Barnard's surgery was received with adulation; in the United States, Shumway nearly ended up being prosecuted. John Hauser, the Santa Clara County coroner, met Shumway with a threat of prosecution. The infringement was that the donor did not have an autopsy performed to confirm that he was dead since performing an autopsy would have ruined the organs for transplantation. Surgeons were being indicted as killers. As a result of this threat of prosecution, organ donations stopped or slowed dramatically. It's like an old Perry Mason TV series where the prosecutor is standing in front of the jury, pointing their index finger at the transplant surgeon while declaring "ladies and gentlemen of the jury, there is your killer."

If we are to use the Pope's language, that death needs to involve "decomposition," "disintegration," and "separation," then it will truly stop all organ transplantation. Without the criterion of brain death, where the organs remain viable, there will be a dramatic deterioration in the quality of organs that can be harvested and transplanted.

According to the World Health Organization, in 2014 120,000 solid organs were transplanted—more than 80,000 kidney, 26,000 liver and 6,500 heart transplants in 93 countries. After Austria, the United States has the highest per capita rate of transplants. Organ transplantation extends lives for a significant number of people.   But we cannot escape the fact that this is made possible by a legal definition of death and not a biological one. If organs are truly dead, they cannot be harvested and brought to life again. It seems that this need for policy to determine death has hindered a more scientific study of death and the dying process.

Science and Death

It does not help that today, because of improvements in medical technology most functions of organs can be replaced by machines. As a result, more opportunities exist to maintain the body alive while being in a state of death. It is becoming more common, especially in industrialized countries, that death has become a medical decision: the decision of whether to keep you on support systems while being "traditionally" dead or to give up and let you die. There is now a choice in some cases, and dying is seen as the last resort when everything else has failed.

Dying has been shunned, and now has become a private and exclusively a clinical catastrophe, often taking place behind a drawn hospital polyester room divider. The body is then transported to the mortuary or funeral home, bathed, dressed with fresh makeup–ready for the living's parody of the final chapter. The expenditure on funeral rites is, of course, for the living. As Dame Cicely Saunders, founder of the hospice movement, said, "How we die remains in the memory of those who live on."

The closest we get to observe death is the study of Near Death Experience. Raymond Moody coined the term Near Death Experience—NDE—as early as 1975. These are people who experienced dying and yet made it back to consciousness. Moody described survivors who 'let go' and accepted their death, but when they survived and gained consciousness, reported experiences of great joy. Although there are exceptions—especially with the use of medications at the end of life—Moody describes how, after travelling through darkness the dying person comes against a bright light, accompanying "beings of light" that helped them review their life. Many people report such experiences across many cultures. The interesting residue after these NDEs is frequently that individuals report having a diminished fear of death.

It was up to a chemistry professor with West Texas A&M to find some of the physiology reasons for NDEs. James E. Whinnery studied fighter pilots who were subjected to extreme gravitational forces in a giant centrifuge. Under extreme g-forces, where blood is pushed away from the brain, fighter pilots experience loss of consciousness, and similar to NDEs, included the tunnel experience and the bright lights. The experience of death, a calming attraction into a bright light, has been described as a "peaceful" experience. With such overwhelming evidence, and many other religious epiphanies that assure us that the passage to the other side is a peaceful and spiritual experience, why are we then so afraid of dying? There is another aspect of death. Not the scientific one but the experiential one. And with this experience, further caricaturized in fiction especially violent films, dying is nothing but peaceful.

Lora-Jean Collett and David Lester made this distinction in 1969 and devised a scale to distinguish between the fear of death from the fear of the process of dying. Some older adults were better at confronting death than others. In an interesting study, James Griffith from Shippensburg University, and his colleagues examined attitudes toward dying and death among older men who had different experiences with danger. The group of men included skydivers (high death risk), nursing home residents (high death exposure), volunteer firefighters (high death risk and high death exposure), and a control group. Their analyses identified that accepting death by risking death reduces the fear of death. High death riskers are better at accepting death. It seems that the fear of death can be minimized, perhaps not only by risking death but also by being exposed to dying people. Can it truly be that we have nothing to fear but fear itself?

Fear of dying not death

Most people have a fear of the dying process. We cannot conceive of a "good" way to die. We might opt for the less gruesome options, but these are not options that we will ever embrace. In one study looking at what people said is their ideal way to die, Gilbert Meilaender from Valparaiso University suggested a one-word answer: Suddenly! The idea is to live as long as possible at the peak of our vigor and then, when the time has come, to die quickly and painlessly. Doubtless he is right about contemporary attitudes toward death. If we have to go, let it be quickly and painlessly. But in truth, dying is likely to be very different. With our advancing and encroaching technology, it is less likely that dying will become a more protracted affair despite our wishes or intentions.

Surprisingly, when we try to hasten the process, we as a society are becoming more sensitive and less accepting of technology helping us to die. In the USA, an older woman, Sharlotte Hydorn, recently gained a measure of notoriety by offering to mail you, for only $60, a package containing GLADD exit bags—Good Life and Dignified Death. The kit included a plastic bag, medical tubing, two canisters of helium and instructions on how to commit suicide—by placing the bag on your head and filling it with helium, which deprives the body of oxygen. The body does not know it is being denied oxygen since the helium mimics oxygen. You die peacefully. Before her death in 2013 in her San Diego home at the age of 93, she was sued for tax evasion and had her property searched by the FBI. Local FBI agents contacted some of her customers. It is important to highlight this ambiguous relationship our society has with death. Especially for older adults, how we say we want to die is frequently quite different from how we deal with death or how we are allowed to deal with our own death. Since more than a quarter of us will likely die in an emergency room, our final departure might look nothing like we envisage. It is likely that it would look more like a chaotic medical soap opera with the whirring of machines and murmured orders given by medical staff. In contrast, our expectation of a dignified release of life, perhaps with Mozart's Requiem Mass in D minor playing in the background appears unlikely to be realized. The availability of "good death" seems to elude us, even when it is available.

Despite the availability of hospice care—both at home and at hospitals, which often involves palliative care targeted to relieve pain, considered the gold standard for end-of-life care—most older adults still experience widespread distress in the final stages of life. We deal with dying underhandedly. In hushed tones, we conspire to give the dying person an answer to their wishes. More than half of the attending physicians admitted to helping AIDs patients die. Overall, more than one in five helped patients terminate their sufferings through the administration of lethal pain medications. In an early survey in 1996 in Michigan, more than half of physicians and two out of three of the general public supported physician-assisted death. In the state of Oregon more than two out of three physicians supported legalizing physician-assisted death, with just under half of the physicians willing to undertake the procedure themselves if asked by their patient.

The religious fervor to curtail this option has not slowed the growing number of states that have legalized physician-assisted death. With six US states and four countries that today openly and legally authorize active assistance in dying of patients, the list of states/countries is growing. Language is important. There is nothing absolute in these situations. Physicians cannot determine with infallible certainty that someone is going to die, sometimes the medication used does not work as intended, or is delayed, the process of taking a pill is sometimes physically impossible, and the idea of injecting a person with enough opioids to kill them is not family friendly and it is killing without consent. These are all valid criticism that poses moral challenges. Whether we define the option as assisted death rather than assisted suicide plays a major role in public's reaction. Language matters because language exposes our fears of being killed. But we are also afraid of dying in agony, which is what assisted death aims to eliminate.

Agonal death

Agony comes from the Greek word "to struggle." The process of dying, especially among frail older adults, is that of a struggle. In the stage right before death, an older person is often accompanied by disorientation, struggling to breathe with long pauses in between loud, labored breaths—called Cheyne-Stokes breathing. Sometimes a death rattle is heard in the breathing when there is liquid in the lungs. Sometimes the person may start convulsing. This agonal process is eloquently described in the *Tibetan Book of the Dead*. Originally composed in the 8th century by Padmasambhava and written down by his primary student Yeshe Tsogyal, it was re-discovered in the 14th century when it became known as *Bardo Thodol* in Tibet. *Bardo Thodol* is a book that describes experiences that our consciousness goes through <u>after</u> death. It is a story of how the soul liberates itself from the transitional stage that is earth. The fight for the soul takes place in the *Bardo*, the interval between death and the next rebirth. Through death, awareness becomes freed from the body. It then creates its own dream by leaving the human world–a dream that can both peaceful and distressing. Not surprisingly, a "white light" is featured in the many stages of *Bardo*. On seeing this white light, if the dead person reacts with joy, then they are saved. In contrast, if they recoil in fear then they will be sucked into hell. The one lesson to take away is to be happy. It is no wonder that such a guidebook to the subconscious formed the basis for the 1964 book *The Psychedelic Experience*—an LSD field guide by the champions of the psychotropic, Timothy Leary, Ralph Metzner and Richard Alpert. The experience of altered consciousness is not exclusively for the dead it seems.

Many of these spiritual interpretations attempt to explain the agonal stage of death–the struggle at the end of life. But medical interpretations may be more useful to us since these explain the likelihood of whether the person is experiencing pain. Especially in the agonal breathing stage—known as dyspnea—labored breathing occurs. At the end of life, dyspnea is defined as an uncomfortable awareness of breathing, breathlessness, shortness of breath, cough, fatigue and gasping–sometimes lasting for weeks or months. Beyond the subjective symptom of dyspnea, the expression of gasping occurs, which can be a brainstem reflex; it is the last respiratory pattern prior to terminal apnoea—when you stop breathing altogether.

Usually a sign of bad amateur theatrics, in real life such final dyspnea is very common among older adults' final release. Such convulsive gasping characterizes the negative experience of watching someone die. Although patients who are gasping are likely unconscious and are not experiencing pain or suffering, we still do not know whether that is the case. Attending physicians explain that endorphins and other natural painkillers are being produced, but we have no confirmation of such likely conjectures because no study exists that confirms this. It is unlikely that they are brain stem dead, or there would be no gasping response. This uncertainty fuels our fear of dying. With more than 151,000 deaths a day throughout the world, it remains a mystery how little we know. Science has yet to help alleviate this fear. Evidence that contradicts that there is no pain at the end-of-life remains forthcoming. Until then, the fear of dying remains real.

Pain and Death

Despite the overwhelming desire to not die in pain, and despite the primary desire for those who are dying in hospital to receive adequate pain and symptom management, most of us will still die in pain. A British study found that over a third of dying patients die in pain. Nearly eight out of every ten hospital-deaths occurred without a palliative care or formal pain management. More than eight out of every ten older long-term care facility residents in the United States experienced untreated or undertreated pain at the time of death. While seven out of ten people who died while on Medicare—a Federal health insurance program mainly for older adults—regardless of their age or where they died, received an inadequate amount of pain management. In response to these prevalent realities Sara Imhof and Brian Kaskie in summarizing their study on pain management at the end-of-life admonished policy makers by stating that: "…we can only conclude that public policies will fall even further behind the advancement of evidence-based pain-policy guidelines, and the number of Americans who continue to suffer needlessly in pain at the time of death will only increase." The near future looks bleak.

Older adults die in many different contexts (e.g., at home, nursing home, hospital, hospice care) resulting in variable pain management. Even though hospice care is the gold standard, very few dying patients and their families take advantage of this option, and when they do they tend to use it too late–two weeks before they die. Pain management is not as straightforward as it seems, especially among people who are either non-responsive or have severe dementia. Other than specific pain brought about from the illness itself, other complications result from the body shutting down. Nausea and vomiting, common features in many advanced diseases, is intensely debilitating. Constipation is common in dying patients because of immobility, poor diet, dehydration, weakness, and some drugs, such as opioids–usually morphine sulphate–used to treat pain. All of these expressions of end-of-life are related in some way. Patients who are close to death often develop audible respiratory secretions—death rattle—caused by the patient's inability to clear the throat normally. As distressing as this sounds, we still do not know what the dying person experiences, or even if they are aware of this. How much of this pain is real—experienced by the patient—and how much is by projected by those witnessing death remains a valid question. Especially with the amount and type of medications that dying patients receive, there is great uncertainty whether pain medication eliminates the pain, eliminates responses to the pain, reduces the awareness of the patient or simply subdues them. These are questions that scientists seem reluctant to examine with dying patients.

Although pain itself remains a very direct experience—a feeling of intense discomfort—the perception is extremely complex. Pain causes adaptive features throughout the body. Thus, the nervous system is operating as a self-organizing arrangement, having a memory that considers pain as beneficial in protecting you. In a sense, in most circumstances–your brain and your body value pain as important safety feedback. Treating pain is a misnomer. Medicating the pain severs the communication between the brain and your body, which is very effective when the pain is short-term. When the pain is long-term the brain has only one alternative, to increase the signal of the communication. The pain will get stronger. The difficulty of treating pain can only be gauged by the epidemic overdose deaths brought by the over-use of opioid pain medication and their cheaper and more accessible variant, heroin. In the United States in 2014, the rate of deaths from opioid overdoses doubled since 2000 with a total of 47,055 drug overdose deaths, representing 14.7 deaths per 100,000 persons. All indications are that this opioid overdose epidemic is worsening. Treating pain, whether through prescribed medication or self-medication, is dangerous, addictive, and by all indications ineffective in the long term. The brain "requires" pain to remain a feedback mechanism in order to protect itself from harm. Our attempts to subdue the feedback by opioids only incite the brain to increase the pain. In the end the brain always wins.

In reality, we have little knowledge about pain during the dying process. That this process remains an enigma highlights the level of ageism that pervades research. The final frontier remains not out of reach but ignored. Despite our psychology's fixation with dying and the associated pain, science seems not interested in death.

Death in Philosophy and Psychology

Death occupies a central theme in philosophy and psychology, especially when addressing our understanding of sense of being, as in metaphysics—a branch of philosophy interested in the first principle of things. Metaphysics asks radical questions about such abstract concepts as being, knowing, substance, cause, identity, time, space and death. Some philosophers tried to educate the public about the irrelevance of worrying about death. But most philosophers misunderstand people's fear, which is not about death (which they cannot know) but the process of dying. Epicurus (341–270), the philosopher who gave us a key tenet of the Constitution—that all people are created equal—writing to Menoeceus invokes: "Death …the most awful of evils, is nothing to us, seeing that, when we are, death is not come, and, when death is come, we are not." Except that he forgot, to his detriment, that dying is a process all by itself. Epicurus suffered from kidney stones. If the stones grow too big they can block the ureter, causing excruciating back pain that radiates to the groin with each episode lasting 20 to 60 minutes. In some cases, the illness induces nausea, vomiting, fever, blood in the urine, pus in the urine, and painful urination. Epicurus finally succumbed to this pain in 270 BC at the age of 72. He might have understood the concept of death correctly, but he learned that dying is a completely different concept.

Other philosophers discuss the morality of death, usually from two very broad camps. On one side is the argument championed by Thomas Nagel, arguing that death is always an evil, since continued life always makes good things happen. The opposing view, spearheaded by Bernard Williams, argues that while premature death is a misfortune, the expectation of death makes us who we are now and forces us to have meaningfully attachment to the present. When Simon Critchley compiled the thoughts of more than 190 philosophers about death, his central theme was the idea that death provides humans with an urgency to live in the present. Our fear of death defines our zest for life.

Death defines Life

The fact that you and I will eventually die and be "no more" is a fact known and understood only by humans, as Jorge Luis Borges reminds us. Although animals have an avoidance of death, they live in the present. They don't comprehend their destiny. Only humans have the capacity to project reality in time and imagine their future. Only humans realize the significance of being "no more" As such, philosophers have stressed the importance of death because it defines our humanity.

Philosophers use the concept of death to define the interactions we have with the present. The expectation of death is the only real aspect of the passage of time. Knowing that we are going to die and be "no longer alive" defines the present as "being alive." Two seminal paradigms changed how we think about ourselves through our concern with death. Starting in the 1900s with Sigmund Freud's psychodynamic theory, where he emphasized the subconscious—a facet of self that is hidden from us. Freud assigned the idea of death itself as a drive—termed *Thanatos*—a name borrowed from the Greek God of death. Then, culminating in the late 1900s, German philosopher Martin Heidegger argued that what separates us from a machine is the empathy to *care*—we take ownership of what we do and feel because we are connected to the fact that we will die. These simplified renditions adequately serve our argument that death is a central fulcrum in philosophical thought.

As with the concept of the Trinity in Catholicism—where three divine persons forming God as one entity—both Freud and Heidegger developed a triptych panorama of the human psyche. Freud developed the *id*—a primitive and instinctive system that embraces Eros, containing our libido and *Thanatos*, our aggressive instinct. The second part is the *ego*—which mediates between the unrealistic id and the external real world according to the reality principle. The third system, *superego*—reflects the values and morals of society consisting of conscience and the ideal self. These three components—the *id*, *ego* and *superego*—dynamically form the three components in the psychodynamic model. While Martin Heidegger developed a philosophy based on our perception of time and our own voyage through this time. The triptych he developed is based on temporal dimensions: *past* (thrownness/disposedness), *future* (projection/ understanding), and *present* (fallen-ness/fascination). We are on a continuum of time that will end. This is what Heidegger famously calls "being-towards-death". Heidegger needed death in order for us to care to own our life rather than just living it.

In both these seminal philosophies, it is important to appreciate that the idea of death forms a central theme. Michel de Montaigne said this much better: "The premeditation of death is the premeditation of liberty; he who has learned to die has unlearned to serve." This anxiety about dying is why we care—we feel responsible for our lives. It is the primary fulcrum that energizes human engagement in a world that we own, that is personal and not a backdrop for a theatrical existence. Surprisingly although philosophers place the intuitive knowledge of death at the center of our sense of being, our psychology refutes it outright.

Death remains an important lynch pin when constructing theories about how people behave because death—our understanding of death—means that we start to care about our world, our behavior and existence. All philosophers have discussed death, some in passing others in more detail. However, Heidegger's interpretation most strongly emphasizes the central nature of our death belief. He argues that our knowledge that we will die forms an appreciation of our ultimate non-existence and that our time is fleeting. This makes us aware of our temporality, our time limit. Without this appreciation, we would not have a sense of involvement. Freud's and Heidegger's interpretation suggest that a developmental process exists in that our appreciation of our own demise translates directly to our caring–to us owning our world and doing something about it. Science has provided some surprising support for this interpretation.

Reminders of death: Mortality Salience

More than five decades ago, the British psychologist Sylvia Anthony reported that children are troubled by the idea of death at a very young age. In Ernest Becker's 1973 Pulitzer Prize-winning nonfiction work, *The Denial of Death*, argues that all human action is taken to ignore or avoid the anxiety generated by the inevitability of death. Death seems central to our psychology. The anxiety results from having two opposing and contradictory ideas together, known as cognitive dissonance. On one hand, we want to become engaged with life and think of ourselves as a meaningful part of the world. On the other hand, what does anything matter anyway if we ultimately become "no more"—if all this wonderment we call life is but a temporary sensation?

According to Becker, people spend their entire lives trying to make sense of these conflicting thoughts. We are so afraid of death that we deny death by creating alternate realities. Realities where we will not "cease to be." We take comfort in the fact that others share this alternate reality. Of course, Becker is referring to religion.

This idea found a home when three psychologists used it as the basis for what they called Terror Management Theory (TMT). In *The worm at the core: On the role of death in Life*, authors Sheldon Solomon, Jeff Greenberg, and Tom Pyszczynski argue that the terror of death forms a core personality strategy that drives us to manage it by developing and supporting an elaborate social world order, where we delude ourselves by diminishing the finality of death. The title of this book expounds on the William James assertion that knowledge of death is the 'worm at the core' of human existence. This social construction includes a world that is orderly according to some belief system: That humans strive for meaning and validity in life largely to counteract their fear of death. This process is strong enough that being reminded of death—yours or someone else's—results in an over-reaction to buttress those beliefs that pacify death–an *existential anxiety buffer*. Death reminds us to care about the world and to protect our beliefs. By providing information about death, we subsequently hold on to our beliefs more forcefully. Fear of death makes us hold to our beliefs as a security blanket.

Hundreds of studies support this prediction. The classic study occurred with a group of judges who were divided into two groups, with one group having subtle reminders of death contained in the questions (mortality salience group). Both groups were then asked to review the case history of a hypothetical prostitute and to suggest a bail bond amount in dollars. The group with mortality salience came down harshly on the hypothetical prostitute, assigning an average bond of $455, while the control group averaged only $50. But this mortality salience generalizes to other aspects of our moral behavior–even political views. By asking participants to write about either their own death (the mortality salience group) or a control topic and then presenting them with someone who wrote disparagingly about their political views and gave them the opportunity to choose the amount of hot sauce the target would have to consume. As predicted by TMT, participants who were reminded of their death allocated a particularly large amount of hot sauce to their worldview-threatening target. But this is not just about punishing prostitutes or punishing people with hot sauce.

Our awareness of death strengthens our negative feelings toward others who are different. We increase the distance between "us" and "them". The authors expose how this fear of death dictates our day-to-day behavior. "Social" priming—being made aware of certain characteristics such as being a professor, death, money, ethnicity, rudeness, being older, consumer choices, voting as well as words, pictures and other cues—results in changes to our attitude and subsequently changes how we behave. Making us more conservative. It is not surprise therefore, that such a radical, powerful and pervasive prediction was surrounded by controversy. In the final analysis, the overall contention is unchallenged: Certain cues prime our attitude that influences our behavior.

Because it is very easy to create mortality salience— just mentioning death or asking questions about death can create the condition—it can be abused or manipulated. There are many examples of such abuse. The top concern of Americans is terrorism, although a Washington Post article by Andrew Shaver in November 2015 titled "You're more likely to be fatally crushed by furniture than killed by a terrorist" highlights the misplaced fear we have. Fear is manipulated. Psychologists interpret human culture as a belief system constructed to explain and give meaning to life and to resist confronting death.

This fear can be dealt with in two ways. The first is to deal very harshly with anything or anyone that reminds us of the threat of death. Anyone that is associated with death (e.g. terrorist) will be more severely punished than similar people or items that do not (e.g. furniture). We are not afraid of cars that kill the equivalent of a planeload full of passengers every day, yet we are afraid of airplanes. Fear is irrational and malleable.   The second strategy is to diminish the permanence of death. That somehow, even after death, we will still be around. Such tricks of psychology include a belief in heaven or reincarnation (either literally or symbolically)–or to establish a more enduring presence even after your death, such as legacy (statues, books, art, street names).

Our concern with death, consciously and subconsciously, determines how we conduct our life. Our morbid fear of dying, dying in pain is further promoted in the news. Portraying terrifying individual cases of trauma. This fear of dying elevates death as more than a state of non-being. Thinkers like Freud and Heidegger used our fear of death to build theoretical models explaining their concept of living. This brings us back to the beginning: Death defines our strategy for living. Other than the process of dying, which remains mired in moral judgments and scientific ignorance, death remains an important psychological foundation for us without really knowing why. Other than experiments showing the effectiveness of the fear of death in changing our behavior, we remain in the dark as to why this should be so. This is truly a new frontier for science.

One solution is to keep fear from controlling your life by confronting your own mortality. Once you accept that life is ethereal, than you can live an authentic life. We have come full circle discussing what the Epicureans and the Stoics preached more than two centuries ago. But can we confront our mortality in the face of death defined as a medical failure. This personal enlightenment remains out of reach for most people. Despite the importance of the "concept" of death, it seems that humans cannot come to grips with death. Even when someone close to us dies, we hold on to shreds of belief about their continued existence in realms that are independent of us. This vestige of residual existence exists throughout all religions. The belief in immortality, however flamboyant this seems in the sharp light of logic, seems a perfect way to diminish the fear of death, albeit for the short term.

Death, the Final Frontier: Conclusion

Of all disciplines, biologists perhaps gain an advantage in accepting death not only as a natural process but also as a necessary process. Death is detrimental to the individual, but necessary for the species to develop. Biologists understand death because they look at species and how species develop. Within the cycle of new generations, slight changes and adaptation, death plays a positive and central role. It is a way of reshuffling the cards to get a better deal. That higher turnover (death rate) means that the species is more adaptive—this is known as r-selection. The alternative biological strategy would be to have fewer offspring but to invest more into their nurturing, and humans constitute a K-selection species. Biologists have become so good at dealing with death that they categorize species on the basis of their death rate.

For humans, with a bigger brain, comes self-reflection and ushers in a frightening awareness. We see death very differently from biologists. Any control we might have in the process remains contested by religious beliefs—morality translated into civil laws. It seems that religious belief protects death as a sacred passage. But when the passage of death is protracted and painful, realistic questions exist about the humanity of these beliefs. The primal fear we have of death contrasts with the crucial role death plays in our survival as a species. Death remains central to any theory of humankind, from philosophy, psychoanalysis, to psychology. Its importance remains unchallenged but somewhat perplexing. One possible explanation emerges from our survival strategy. Our K-strategy, to nurture a few children and to be able to impart knowledge and protection requires that we have a big brain that can collect all that knowledge and achieve the longevity to be around to impart what we have learned. However, there was an additional consequence. Humans become self-aware, and the first shock is knowing that we will die. The primordial fear of death was one of the consequences of a larger brain and increased longevity. This is the price we pay for longevity, and it has repercussions in our psychology.

The search for immortality contrasts with living longer. Although scientists delude us by assuming that living longer will eventually lead to immortality, or close to a state of immortality, our psychology will accept nothing less than not dying. Immortality is not a scientific endeavor, it is a psychological crutch that we rely on to dispel our fear of death. Some scientists rely on our confusion when they sell immortality and talk about "longer, healthier life." But immortality is different. We do not want to die healthy we just do not want to die. The benefits of longer life exposes the predicament of when is a good time to die? Would living up to 150 years of age help alleviate our fear of dying? And the answer is no. Peddling hope that immortality is within reach is not cruel, we demand scientists to maintain this illusions on our behalf.

---∞---

Chapter 7

Delusional Life

"To wisely live your life, you don't need to know much
Just remember two main rules for the beginning:
You better starve, than eat whatever
And better be alone, than with whoever."

Omar Khayyám, *Rubaiyat*

F ear of death is a price we pay for our species'
strategy for survival. A bigger brain results in
increased longevity, but also results in self-
awareness.   Throughout this exploration of immortality,

from genes to biology to lessons from life from the masters of extreme longevity themselves—Centenarians—a consistent theme emerges. That theme is the importance of our history and our environment, and that everything around us is connected. Even our strategy for survival has consequences. When combined, those two components— our history and our environment—form the basis for explaining our biological life, including our longevity, better than any other aspect of our life. The final conclusion that we have taken from this journey is that the single purpose for our existence is to ensure that we match our environment so that we can survive and thrive and pass on our genes. There is no other higher calling. We are here in order to survive, learn and pass on acquired survival skills. It seems that this strategy allows for our immortality genes to continue on their path to infinity. Longevity is a part of this strategy—an important part because it comes with the omnibus package of health. Longevity is inseparable from health. But in our psychology, immortality holds a very different meaning.

Stephen Cave, in his excellent book *Immortality*, organizes his thoughts about how humans aim to achieve immortality under four main narratives: Staying alive, Resurrection, Soul and Legacy. All of these are mental tricks for humans to accept immortality or at the very least, to deny the concept of death. The Soul's legacy in immortality is that at death our soul separates from the body and at some point, is (re)united in heaven or hell. The Christian and Muslim belief is that at some point, the perfect body will again reunite with the soul.

Stephen Cave reminds us of Jorge Luis Borge's quote that "Except for man, all creatures are immortal for they are ignorant of death." As humans, our capacity for delusion is unfathomable. Perhaps such trickery and cleverness could be the original sin that got humans evicted from the cerebral Garden of Eden. What distinguishes us from other animals is not carnal knowledge but the awareness that we will die. Such knowledge dispels the belief that we live in an idealized world—where nothing changes and we are safe—to a reality that is hard, uncompromising and random, eventually ending in death. We will no longer exist. But we only know of death intellectually. As Freud wrote in 1915 "It is indeed impossible to imagine our own death." Which is why children believe in immortality from early on in their life. Death disrupts an idealized world that we carry with us in our brain—a world where we are in control and where bad things happen to bad people only. Death disrupts this perfect order and is the ultimate witness to our faulty perception of the world. This explains why when people are reminded of their mortality they tend to cling more fiercely to their existing beliefs. Religious belief is a pushback against the reality of death. Our fear of death is so strong that it dictates human behavior.

Terror Mis-Management

A whole industry exists that manages our daily information. This is not a sophisticated conspiracy but a managed system of information engrained in our institutions. Sociologists have examined this phenomenon for more than a century. Institutions formulate beliefs. Our belief that we are immortal, whether by having a Soul, or by other delusional tricks that we can stay Alive, Resurrection and Legacy. These strategies of Terror Management Theory, as eloquently discussed by Stephen Cave, are not exclusive and can be used together or in sequence. When one strategy ultimately fails to deny death, we adopt the next strategy in sequence. Hopefully we die before we run out of our delusional choices. We have delusional strategies in order to rationalize—diminish—the reality of death, and then we practice strategies that minimize death—risk behaviors for example—that might not protect us. Surrounded by our own psychology to deny death, we focus on events that are unlikely, dramatic and sensational. By focusing on these aspects of dying (i.e. in a plane crash) we divert our attention from what would most likely kill us—the stress of worrying about dying in a plane crash.

How we really die

Not all healthy people live long lives. We acknowledge that being healthy and staying alive are two different constructs. There are many ways to die other than through ill-health. In 2016 Martin Makary and Michael Daniel with Johns Hopkins University, revealed that after analyzing deaths over an eight-year period in the U.S., more than 250,000 deaths per year are due to medical error. This figure surpasses the U.S. Centers for Disease Control and Prevention's third leading cause of death—respiratory disease, which kills close to 150,000 people per year. Medical intervention is the third killer in the U.S.

Such deaths are known as iatrogenic, a word that comes from Greek for *iatros*, "healer" and *genesis*, "origin". Ivan Illich, the Austrian philosopher, popularized the concept of Iatrogenesis when he wrote *Medical Nemesis: The Expropriation of Health* in 1976. It is difficult to assess the extent of iatrogenic deaths in countries where data is not so rigorously collected. Most medical errors are also not due to inherently bad health care workers, but represent systemic problems such as inadequate management of patients and their medications. But these deaths do highlight a behavioral component of dying other than one's health. In addition to iatrogenic disease, there are other behavioral causes of death.

In 2014 in the U.S., cigarette smoking accounted for more than 480,000 deaths, drinking too much alcohol was responsible for 88,000 deaths, more than half of which were due to binge drinking. In 2011, more than half of adults aged 18 years or older were considered physical lazy, refraining from physical activity. In most cases, luck also plays a role. We cannot do very much with luck. Jean Calment, the longest living human lived to see her 122th birthday, outlived her daughter Yvonne who died of pneumonia and her grandson Frédéric who died of a motorcycle accident. Both died at the age of 36. We might have great potential for longevity but we cannot completely control the environment, we can only minimize the randomness of accidents. Among centenarians, randomness also plays a role in their death.

A 2016 report by Jiaquan Xu of CDC's National Center for Health Statistics shows that between 2000 and 2014, death rates for centenarians increased 33% for unintentional injuries. Having lived for a century, evaded most diseases that brought down most of your family and friends, what kills you in the end might be a wet floor in the bathroom, a small rug in the hallway, or an inattentive walk across the kitchen to nibble on that last donut in the middle of the night.

In truth, only one real cause of death exists—oxygen starvation to the brain. The cause of death listed on death certificates is really the cause of the cause. As simple as this might seem, formalizing a definition of death has never been easy. Sherwin Nuland, an American surgeon, has made the point that death in older age is often a protracted affair rather than a clear-cut process. He quotes an elderly patient as saying, "Death keeps taking little bits of me." For older adults, the final chapter is a death knell that starts with faint tinkle bells of biological failures that crescendo into a biological implosion of the body.

Throughout this book, these external factors comprise the Makeham effect–referring to constant environmental threat of death. This constant varies by country, which is why life expectancy is higher in industrialized countries. Clean water, safe environments, restricted wars, vaccinations, adequate shelter, good standards of living, health care and education all diminish the threat of death from the environment. This is no small feat as death statistics by iatrogenesis and unintentional injuries still appear. If we truly want people to live longer, the most logical approach would be to completely eliminate this threat from our environment.

Such an approach is nuanced, long term, and latent. It is not sexy to promote health when the results take a generation to emerge. It takes years for any progress to be recorded. Whoever initiates such a long-term strategy needs to forego any personal adulation. The search for immortality can take many forms, most of which are not exclusive. Achieving notoriety or enhancing your legacy is another way of achieving some sense of immortality. But for this, you must receive individual recognition. If individual recognition is what we desire, what could be more earth-shatteringly good than to cure diseases? Most often when scientists are asked why they want to extend their life span (they never say they are after immortality), they say they want to cure disease. They want to eliminate suffering. Psychologically this is logical, but in reality the argument is flawed.

Eliminating all diseases

What if we eliminated the top diseases of older adults? Goodbye cancer, diabetes, cardiovascular disease, stroke, influenza pneumonia, and chronic obstructive lung disease.

Can we then live forever, as some have suggested? The surprising answer is that curing all of these diseases will result in very little change in additional life. Of course, we can only do this statistically.

Kenneth Manton and his colleagues from Duke University eliminated one disease at a time in their statistical modeling. They found that if we eliminate all of these killer diseases, then overall we expect to see those over 87 years of age to live an additional 5.7 years for males (estimated for 1987) and 6.5 years for females. This is about the same as improvement in life expectancy at 65 in the last 100 years in the USA (5.7 years). If you are 65 years old today, you have a 50/50 chance of living an additional 5.7 years than if you were living in the 1900s. In the last hundred years, the great improvement in life expectancy is not among older adults, but among newborns and infants. It has very little to do with clinical care at later ages.

However, this is not the end of the story.

Most older adults suffer from not just one, but multiple health conditions. If we assume that we can cure one disease–say cancer–we will still be faced, sooner rather than later, with another disabling disease that might kill us more slowly and perhaps more painfully.

Douglas G. Manuel with the Institute for Clinical Evaluative Sciences in Toronto, Canada, and his colleagues calculated what happens when they eliminated specific killer diseases from their data. They predicted that by eliminating cancer, one fifth of the years of life gained would be spent in poor health—and increased cost. On the other hand, eliminating musculoskeletal conditions would result in a year of good health for women and less than half a year for men. Logically it would be better to cure musculoskeletal conditions then cancer. But that might not catch on. As a society we focus on the obvious and the salient that stands in our way of developing an effective public health strategy for managing ill health at older ages.

As life expectancy has increased, the number of healthy years lost to disability has also increased in most countries. Joshua Salomon from the Harvard School of Public Health and his colleagues found that although most countries have made substantial progress in reducing mortality over the past two decades, non-fatal disease and injury have not improved to the same degree.

Our progress in health outcomes is also slowing down in the US, especially diseases that we can control and especially for women. Nearly 20 years ago, the United States was closer to the middle rank of industrialized countries, but countries like Ireland and South Korea improved sharply, leaving the United States behind. In addition, across all industrialized countries, because we are living longer and living with diseases, the occurrence of chronic diseases has increased. Finding a cure should be matched with finding care. Our reliance on medical breakthroughs ignores the immediate need that we face. We need to think about finding care as much as finding a cure. But then where is the individual adulation? The search for immortality is about individual adulation. It's about pampering an ego that cannot accept that it is mortal. It is about being recognized. If curing disease remains problematic, what else can be done to provide a sense of personal victory over death? What would be better still? The answer again comes back to treating aging as a disease. Let's deal with aging.

Slowing Biological Aging vs. Curing All Diseases:

In 2013 in an issue of Health Affairs, Dana Goldman with the University of Southern California and her team of policy analysts, epidemiologists and economists, ran a simulation of the benefits of slowing aging compared to curing disease. Of course, this is akin to having an economist look at cancer and then coming up with the best solution not to get cancer in the first place. In this case, these pragmatists decided that investing in delaying aging would have a much greater impact on life expectancy than investing in curing diseases directly, a circular argument. If people stop dying early we can increase how long they live. The delusion tricks of immortality are at it again. But aging is not a disease.

An investment in delayed aging would increase the number of healthy older adults by 11.3 million by 2060. But investing in curing fatal diseases of aging would not. Trying to sell aging as a disease is easy. Although no one defines aging accurately and they define "delayed aging" as spending a larger proportion of one's life in good health, free from frailty and disability seems inane. Especially if we consider that they propose delaying aging ". . . by manipulating genes, altering reproduction, reducing caloric intake, modulating the levels of hormones that affect growth and maturation, and altering insulin-signaling pathways." (p. 1699).

Some people believe that we are close to a solution, but maybe not in their lifetime. What to do? The theme of our delusional strategies is to deny us awareness of the finality of death. Perhaps a solution will emerge, a cure in the future. Perhaps we are just born too early. What if we can literally stop the death clock from ticking. Not surprisingly, humans have figured out a way of selling that strategy as well.

Cryonics/ Cryogenics

When Robert Ettinger, a Michigan college physics teacher, wrote *The Prospect of Immortality* in 1964, the research gerontologist Gerald J. Gruman wrote in the preface that he was reminded of Benjamin Franklin when he was shipwrecked. After being rescued, while expressing his feelings of gratitude and thanks, he was asked if he intended to build a chapel to memorialize his safety. "No, indeed not," he replied, "I'm going to build a lighthouse!" Ettinger proposed to build such a pragmatic lighthouse for the dead. By ignoring the reality that all of us will eventually be shipwrecked against our own mortality, Ettinger writes "But with good luck, the manifest destiny of science will be realized, and the resuscitated will drink the wine of centuries unborn. The likely prize is so enormous that even slender odds would be worth embracing." (p.16). He has become the first suspended client of Cryonics Institute and the "manifest destiny of science" holds his legacy under frozen suspended animation.

Cryonics is low-temperature preservation of animals and humans, with the hope of resuscitation in the future. The belief in hope for resurrection is alive and well in the United States and Russia. Three cryonics service providers exist: Alcor Life Extension Foundation Inc. (Arizona, USA), Cryonics Institute (Michigan, USA), and KrioRus (Moscow, Russia). Cryopreservation is becoming increasingly popular. Alcor has enrolled more than 1,000 patients already (2015). Cryonics lists more than 100 (2013), while KrioRus reports more than 50 patients (2015). Although most are from the Russian Federation and the USA (with Californians being the primary clients), more than 100 international clients have registered from all over the world. Under current law, a patient must be legally dead before being cryogenically preserved–usually within 15 minutes of death.

These warehouses store bodies upside down, in liquid nitrogen, in various state of disassembly, under suspended death through freezing. Because ice crystals damage cells, modern methods—and they vary—includes vitrification at -196°C. In vitrification—which means to turn into glass but in this case, slows the cells in a state of animation—more than 60% of the water inside cells is replaced with DMSO (dimethyl sulfoxide), propylene glycol, and a colloid. This completely prevents freezing during deep cooling. Recent experiments have managed to reverse this process in mice—de-vitrified and survived—so the science is improving. Pets can also be cryopreserved. But it is humans who are the main customers. Although prices vary KrioRus reports that a full body cryopreservation costs $36,000 while the brain will cost $12,000. Alcor charges about $125,000 for whole-body suspensions, while just the head will cost you $50,000.

The logic of freezing a dead body in the hope that someday a cure will be found that compels future generations to re-animate you is faulty. What might seem logical on paper is acted out differently in reality.

Freezing Jefferson

Let's assume that you are related to Thomas Jefferson, an author of the American Declaration of Independence who later served as the third President from 1801 to 1809. No greater historical figure exists in the United States. Let's also assume that when he died in 1826 he was able to freeze himself in a state of animation—cryonics. We also need to assume that we could cure him of whatever killed him at age 83 and hopefully also we could ease his constant migraines. Even with modern medicine, this is unlikely to be the case as he likely had prostatic cancer, suffered from chronic bouts of diarrhea, was in the later stages of kidney failure and had pneumonia–things that would kill you to this day. But for the sake of our argument, lets assume that Jefferson is in a state of cryonics and we have the ability to bring him back alive and cure him of all his ailments. This is the ideal vision that Robert Ettinger sold. Let's examine the reality from that ideal.

He wrote numerous manuscripts and books about his personal musings and philosophies. He was a polymath–a scholar of languages, music, philosophy and art. He was a great diplomat, an ideal candidate to preserve for prosperity. But let's bring this into more current focus. Jefferson considered himself to be a "benevolent" slave owner. He considered himself a liberal landowner, and believed that protecting the interest of the common folk protected his interest in a society that allowed him to accrue wealth. He was a real Renaissance man.

Fast forward 200 years and you have the key to bring him alive. We know he had a number of children with his wife, and then when she died, with one of his slaves, a half-sister to his dead wife (fathered by his wife's father). Lets assume that you are one of his descendants living in the United States right now.

Maybe Jefferson needs 24/7 care–changing of diapers, feeding, personal care. He will certainly need full physiotherapy for years assuming that his muscles did not atrophy. He might also quickly become infected with new bacteria and viruses that did not exist in his time. Remember how a new smallpox virus wiped out American Indians on the Trail of Tears. Perhaps he will not be able to survive the new bacteria that surround us today. He might need to be isolated and segregated from the general public. Perhaps he will get a cultural shock, looking at today's U.S. Congress. He will definitely feel sad looking at all the destruction and wars in which we are currently involved. Will he complain about Congress? Will he be labeled as "fake news?" Will he complain about our political direction and endanger an alternate? Will he tell me how to run my business? Perhaps he was slightly eccentric before freezing himself for prosperity. How sane is someone who thinks they are so important for humanity that they would freeze themselves for prosperity? Perhaps the idea that he was important enough for people to recognize his worth in the future was an indication that he was delusional, egoistical, even psychotic. Do we need more politicians? Perhaps being in a frozen state for 200 years played with his internal narrative, so that now that he is free from an internal solitary confinement he might have some psychological issues with reality. Perhaps his brain was really alive for 200 years. Perhaps he was in solitary limbo, without any stimulation—a reduced stimulation frozen bath. Perhaps he would change his will and testament and write you off once he is reanimated. Or perhaps in those 200 years of solitude he has come up with a totally transformative philosophy that will benefit human kind for centuries. Perhaps.

So, the question to you now, to rephrase the San Francisco detective Harry Callahan in the 1971 film *Dirty Harry*, is:

"…you've gotta ask yourself one question: 'Do I feel lucky?' Well, do ya, punk?"

Cryonics is not a way of preserving yourself for prosperity. Think about who will thaw you out and what their motives might be. What is so important about you that someone in the future cannot obtain from the current population, or from other similarly cryogenic optimists? What we have come across is not a logical option but a psychological crutch to keep people from accepting the finality of death. This is not new or as unique as we believe. Unfortunately, California now pays more than $636 million a year to keep dead people alive.

Vent farms

Walking through a sub-acute unit, you notice the sedating quietness and the soft pulsating rhythm of ventilators. Sharp fluorescent lights contrast with the quiet immobility of patients in their guardrail beds. These are comatose patients kept alive. In California, more than 4,000 long-term comatose patients are kept alive on machines. Although some might recover, special units exist where not one of these patients will ever recover. These sub-acute units are referred to as "vent farms," referring to the many ventilators needed to keep all the patients breathing. Vent farms are usually stand-alone, separate units that cater to people who will not recover but who are kept alive because their family or friends refrain from acknowledging that they are dead. Most are private, for-profit organizations, but the cost is borne by the public.

In California, although none of these patients will ever gain consciousness, they are kept alive at a state cost of an average of $900 a day. In 2013, the total cost to the state of California alone came to more than $636 million. California refrains from keeping more accurate figures. This clinical care is provided when there is no chance of improving outcomes. Such costs will continue to increase as the lines between living and dead become more and more blurred, and people become less in tune with the natural course of life that includes death, however untimely. Vent farms are not there for the patients; they are there for the patient's family and friends. The state is paying for the family to delay accepting the death of a loved one. We have come full circle where Lyall Watson's exposition of fear of people being buried alive is replaced with the fear of keeping dead people alive.

There are exceptions. Many other questions remain to this day, including hospitals' use of painkillers and medications given to dying patients, who then present with brain-dead features. Alan Shewmon, Professor of Pediatric Neurology at UCLA Medical School, cites 140 cases of prolonged survival—from a few months to one case of 14 years—by brain-dead patients. Very few patients recover consciousness from being brain dead, apart from a few singular reports of such exceptions. Indeed, scientists who deal with scientific methodology argue that "brain-dead" confuses prognosis with diagnosis. The prognosis that the patient will not regain consciousness is different from the diagnosis that the brain is not functioning. So far, however, despite the variance in how hospitals apply the guidelines for what constitutes death, a declaration of death is not a divisive issue in most industrialized countries. But it can be. Death will emerge as a divisive issue–not because of live donors being killed, but because of the growing number of dead people being kept alive. As with sub-acute units, Vent Farms keep dead people alive solely because the family cannot come to terms with the death of a loved one. It is for the benefit of the living.

As Stephen Cave has enumerated, there are many ways that the living deny that death exists. If you have money you can buy the research. You can tap into the "manifest destiny of science." And if you have a delusional sense of self, surely you can wield science to meet your ambition. Many people do not accept change and if you are used to controlling your environment, you can tailor your life to suite your needs. The rise of oligarchs—extremely rich people—has fueled a new kind of narcissism, the new breed of immortalists.

Oligarchs don't Want to Die

Perhaps the affirmation one gets from being rich—being able to strive to quench any desires, to influence people, modify the world around you—the idea of death seems illogical and unwarranted. A new word has evolved to describe such people, as different from nobility, the ruling class, academics, industry moguls and media stars and these are the oligarchs. Oligarchs synonymous with plutocracy—governance by the wealthy—have come to think that death might be unnecessary, and they are investing money towards abolishing death. They see death as unfair and oligarchs are funding research to find a cure-all—and clever scientists are taking their money. The search is on for the holy grail of biology, a cure for aging. Aging has again become the new frontier that the rich aim to overcome. The most obvious oligarchs are contributing towards this aim by sponsoring anti-aging research. The list below is not exhaustive but provides a comprehensive overview that rich people take dying, and their attempt to evade it, very seriously indeed:

- *The Paul F Glenn Foundation for Medical Research* was founded in 1965 by Paul F. Glenn, with a mission to extend the healthy years of life through research on mechanisms of biology that govern normal human aging and its related physiological decline.
- Founded in 1997 by billionaire Larry Ellison with Kevin Lee as the director of the *Ellison Medical Foundation* is the largest private funder of anti-aging research, spending $45m annually.
- David Murdoch donated $35 million in 2007 to collect health and personal information annually from 11,200 participants—the goal is to reach 50,000 participants—

who also provide one-time urine and blood samples with the hope to find new markers for illnesses such as Alzheimer's disease.

- Since 2009 PayPal cofounder Peter Thiel has been funding Aubrey de Grey's Strategies for Engineered Negligible Senescence (SENS) Research Foundation. SENS funds with about $5m of research annually.

- In 2013 Google announced the creation of *Calico*, short for the California Life Company. Its mission is to reverse-engineer the biology that controls lifespan and "devise interventions that enable people to lead longer and healthier lives." Calico has entered into a joint venture with the pharmaceutical company AbbVie to build a new research facility to investigate age-related diseases, including neuro-degeneration.

- In 2014 Google co-founder Sergey Brin donated nearly $125 million to the *Michael J. Fox Foundation* and $7 million to the *Parkinson's Institute*. Brin has a genetic mutation that sharply raises his risk for Parkinson's. One project is being conducted by 23andMe, co-founded by Brin's separated wife, Anne Wojcicki. The firm scans the DNA submitted by its customers and provides information on their genetic diversity, ancestry, and other traits.

- In 2014, pioneering American biologist and technologist Craig Venter teamed up with the entrepreneur and founder of the X Prize Foundation, Peter Diamandis—announced a new company called *Human Longevity Inc.* Together they are planning to create a giant database of 1 million human genome sequences by 2020, including the genomes of supercentenarians.

- The research project planned by Russian media mogul Dmitry Itskov hopes to interest other billionaires in the

2045 Initiative—named for the target completion date— that will investigate the possibility of transferring the entire content of an individual's brain into a low-cost synthetic brain.

- In 2016 Facebook's Mark Zuckerberg with his wife Priscilla Chan, joined with others to create *Breakthrough Prizes*, which provides funding for scientists who make discoveries that extend human life. Although these are relatively modest $3 million payouts, they are given to six scientists each year.

- David Koch has donated over $400 million to date and $150 million over the coming to numerous institutions involved in cancer research and therapy his biggest donations go towards "moon shot" campaigns to find a cancer cure.

- Johnson & Johnson: $50 million investment deal with the Spanish plasma derivatives giant Grifols—will be based on the discovery that different factors in blood plasma, known as chemokines, can promote or inhibit brain decline.

- Pierre Omidyar, founder of eBay, with his wife Pam Omidyar have donated millions to research on "resiliency," the collective traits that help some individuals bounce back from illness or adversity—but not on aging itself.

- Peter Nygard through *Nygard Biotech* has been promoting somatic cell nuclear transfer (SCNT) essentially cultivating an individual's old stem cells implanted into hollowed-out human eggs, where they multiply. The new and youthful cells, known as autologous stem cells, would then be injected into the original donor. The goal of SCNT is to help cure disease and slow aging. Nygard plans to invest $100 million to build a world-class medical facility in the Bahamas

- The *Buck Institute for Research on Aging* is the only free-standing institute dedicated to age-related research, where Google's *Calico* is based. The institute has been studying ways to inhibit the earliest origins of age-related diseases such as Parkinson's and Alzheimer's disease and has already patented a number of basic findings and technologies.

The search for immortality is driven by an individual desire to deny that death is our only option. The ultimate expression of Terror Management Theory—that you are doing something to diminish the fear of death. All this frantic activity to find the silver bullet that will rid us of death is not for the homeless guy we see every morning as we get our morning cup of coffee, nor is it for those young addicts queuing for their daily free produce, or the young mothers at the WIC clinic downtown. No. The search is for those that have earned their worth. And the reason we can say that with some certainty is that this thinking has created a radical change in our society—a change that has had serious and irreversible repercussions on our health as a nation. We have become divided.

While rich people fund research to find immortality the rest of the population is increasingly dying earlier than we have in the past, and they are dying of amenable diseases—diseases that we can control today. They are sliding down into statistical oblivion, while the rest of us delude ourselves that the search for immortality has benefits for all of us. That such research will trickle down. This is yet another lie that we are willing to ignore to mute our anxiety about our approaching mortality. Poor people are dying at a higher rate while we still believe that we are progressing towards immortality. The quest for immortality, and the advances that we are promoting, does not benefit everyone equally.

Poor People's Life

The life expectancy gap between America's richest 1 percent and its poorest 1 percent is currently slightly over 14 years. In cities, the gap is much wider. Recent figures from the London Health Observatory found the gap in life expectancy, between those in London's affluent and deprived wards, is now nearly 25 years. In the US, the difference between the lowest and the highest 5% in the major cities of New York, Dallas, San Francisco and Phoenix is between 7-13 years. Money talks by determining our lifetime guarantee.

Researchers with Stanford University and MIT, Raj Chetty, Michael Stepner and Sarah Abraham, analyzed 1.5 billion records of individuals aged 40 to 76 years. The results were conclusive. Higher income was associated with greater longevity with the richest and poorest 1% differing by 14.6 years. This inequity is increasing with the rich increasing their life expectancy by around 3 months every year. There was great variability among the poor. Life expectancy for low-income individuals varied substantially across local areas. Then, unexpectedly, we saw this negative trend go national and international.

Between 2014 and 2015 a sudden spike in death showed up in national reports. No one expected this increase in deaths. People started dying earlier. Not by much–maybe 2 or 3 months earlier, but the finding was significant. The first wave of national statistics was quickly followed by questions as to why. The first explanation related to local conditions, blaming the local economic or weather conditions. It then emerged that this increase was not just a national event but also an international phenomenon. Most industrialized countries showed a similar spike in death but for different population groups. This increase in death was global. The surprising detail that came out of all these countries mortality was that the increase in death seems to affect primarily older and specific younger adult populations. With some exceptions, however, older people were dying earlier than at previous years. Small but significant increases in early death among older adults were occurring throughout industrialized countries.

For example, according to the Russian State Statistics Service (Rosstat), in the first quarter of 2015 death rate grew by 5.2 percent compared to the same period last year, with a 22 percent rise in the death rate among those suffering from respiratory illnesses, followed by diseases of the digestive system (10 percent), infectious diseases (6.5 percent), and blood circulation disorders (5 percent). Meanwhile, infant death and death from murder and suicide were falling. One of the clues for this increased death was that respiratory diseases caused by common cold, flu and pneumonia brought about most of the deaths.

In the United States, Anne Case and Angus Deaton wrote about the long-term increase specifically for one group of Americans, White adults. Although from 1978 to 1998, the mortality rate for US Whites aged 45–54 fell by 2% per year on average—which matched the average for other industrialized countries—after 1998, while other industrialized countries continued to show a 2% annual decline in mortality, in the US the 45-54 age group showed half a percent annual increase. There was a marked increase in death of middle-aged White men and women in the United States between 1999 and 2013, reversing decades of progress in lowering mortality. For three groups in particular–those aged (with highest mortality first) 45-49, 56-59 and 50-54. Among American older adults, mortality held constant or improved over this period. This increase for Whites largely resulted from drug and alcohol poisonings, suicide, and chronic liver diseases, including cirrhosis, and was especially severe for those with less education.

Ill health in the United States is locked to our income. And it is not just a matter of throwing money at the problem. For example, maternal death rates are twice that of our neighbors in Canada, despite the fact that we pay twice as much on health care than Canadians. Americans get a very poor return for their health care contribution. The increase in death reflected an underlying decline in self-reported health, mental health and ability to conduct activities of daily living. Furthermore, there was an increase in reports of chronic pain and inability to work, as well as clinically measured deteriorations in liver function. All these indicators point to growing distress in this White population. Although some methodological criticisms exist, such as age adjustment as populations change—the central thesis is robust, that in the USA middle-aged Whites have higher mortality increases than other populations. Surprisingly, this increase is still growing.

Across the Atlantic in the United Kingdom, 2015 saw the largest rise in the number of recorded deaths in England and Wales in more than a decade. Although higher mortality peaked during winter, it remained slightly above the five-year average for the rest of the year. By 2016, mortality was recorded at around 3.8% above the five-year average, but again without accounting for population age changes. This increase was driven largely by increased mortality in over-75-year-olds (83% of the increase). The cause is ascribed to dementia and respiratory diseases, including colds, flu and pneumonia. A similar increase was experienced in many other European countries. It is normal for mortality to peak during winter season, especially for older populations—older adults are more prone to cold weather—but it is not only cold weather that was killing older adults. In Europe, in July 2016, a slight increased mortality among elderly in all countries appeared, the most significant being in France and Portugal since the beginning of July–increases which started during hot months.

We need to be cautious about extrapolating from single-year data or using single methodologies, as this might just be an errant fluctuation. Some spikes in mortality occur frequently, but because this is so consistent across many countries this reversal in life expectancy warrants attention.

Some researchers have argued that social status/class played a role in the increase in deaths–especially in the US, where the spike in deaths occurred among less educated White residents. The downturn in the economy after 2008—although it affected minorities more severely than Whites—was dramatic and unexpected. Minorities have had some time to become acclimatized to this depression. This argument, that sudden onset of poverty, seems to be supported by other data, especially from the U.K.

The U.K. mortality spike occurred in all areas of the country except for London. Since these increased deaths are primarily caused by influenza and pneumonia—the main killers for older adults—environmental factors might also be at play that exacerbates poverty. Although we should see a growing increase in deaths because our population is aging, these yearly fluctuations might be worsened by an increase in both the prevalence of bacteria and viruses and our reduced resiliency to these new infections.

Global climate change and less effective antibiotics–together with a more vulnerable population, which is older and perhaps less resilient because of poverty—might accelerate deaths.   Again, although small, these shifts in trends are unique enough to warrant serious monitoring. The reversal of a half-century of progress in life expectancy might herald a new way of looking at diseases that embraces a more central public health role. We might see that to better address health, we might have to better address economic issues and the environment. The balance that we have enjoyed over the last 50 years might be swinging back and eroding longevity advantages. This might also reflect the growth in centenarians. Global climate change might dramatically affect micro-organisms, which in turn might affect our microbiota causing unforeseen changes to disease.

Conclusion

What is a good age to die? If we push the age of death to 200 years will we be happy then? The answer is, of course, no. The concept of death is abhorrent to us. Death is inconsistent with our belief system that the world is just and consistent. This is the ultimate role of our large brain—it develops a model of reality, one that is perfect and causal, in order to be able to predict our environment. Through a learning process we refine this model in our brain. The construct of death negates this perfect model and we try and refute it. The belief in immortality is just one form of delusional tricks to do just that.

Taking charge of this fear allows us to define what we want to do with our life. *Carpe diem*, the popular Latin saying "seize the day," from the Roman poet Horace's work Odes (23 BC) is defined by the knowledge that we will die. If we had immortality would we truly seize the day? Will we simply waste time since it is so abundant? In this interpretation, death has a positive psychological meaning in our lives. Martin Heidegger positioned the construct of death as the single feature that makes us human. The knowledge that we will die allows us to own and take responsibility for our life. Without this knowledge, we are simply actors in a play. Some people experience a resistance to accept the importance of death and to negate it. As a result, there increasing negative social inequities exist in how we manage our health systems. Instead of providing care, we aim for a cure. The scientific collusion is the final bastion of the delusion of immortality.

However the immortalists argue that the science they are promoting can someday help people. By eradicating disease and eliminating pain, research conducted while searching for immortality will eventually help people. Such concessions might be accepted if it was not for the fact that every year between 2 million to 12 million people will die from water-related disease, most of those are small children struck by virulent but preventable diarrheal diseases. In the developing world 1.1 billion people remain without access to safe water, and 2.6 billion lack adequate sanitation. Water-related diseases are claiming the lives of 5,000 children a day. Not having safe water is second biggest killer of children worldwide, after acute respiratory infections like tuberculosis. We have to ask ourselves about the seriously of our concern to eliminate disease and pain for the majority of the world's population. The involvement of oligarchs, who made large amount of money in careers not related to caring professions or health, to all of a sudden gain an interest in helping people, remains difficult to take seriously. Especially after gaining some knowledge about how to eliminate some of the main killers in the world.

Immortality is a rich person's game and a poor person's delusion. The general public accepts these concessions, that research on immortality will eventually help them, because it helps them subdue that own personal fear of mortality by providing some hope, however irrational such hope might be. In our thinking, we try to believe in constancy in the world. Whenever unforeseen events happen we attempt to either blame it as an erratic event or to consolidate it into our worldview. The reality is that we are always changing and the consistency that we would like the world to exhibit resides more in our thinking than in reality. Immortality holds a prominent role in our consistency worldview. Dealing with immortality we have to dismantle this model of constancy and replace it with a reality that is more fluid and ever changing. Only then can we discard immortality and look at longevity under a different light.

————————————∞————————————

Chapter 8

Future of Immortality

"Let's consider your age to begin with — how old are you?'
'I'm seven and a half exactly.'
'You needn't say "exactly,"' the Queen remarked: 'I can believe
it without that. Now I'll give you something to believe. I'm just one
hundred and one, five months and a day.'
'I can't believe that!' said Alice.
'Can't you?' the Queen said in a pitying tone. 'Try again: draw
a long breath, and shut your eyes.'

– Carroll, L. (1917). *Through the looking glass: And what*
Alice found there. Rand, McNally. p. 88-89

How Old Are You? Unlike the Queen in the Alice in Wonderland story, we are *exactly* as young as Alice herself. Seriously. All of us are just under 11 years old. A crude average of most of our body organs averages about 11 years old. Our biological age is 11 years old. Jonas Frisen, a stem cell biologist at the

Karolinska Institute in Stockholm developed a method for determining the age of each organ. Although some cells remain with us the duration of our life—neurons of the cerebral cortex, cells of your inner lens in our eyes, muscle cells of your heart—the rest of our body engages in in a constant frenzy of change and rejuvenation–a microcosm of death and rebirth across the 37.2 trillion cells that make up our body.

Even our brain changes and renews itself. Joseph Altman first discovered brain cell regeneration—or neurogenesis—in 1962. Recently, Elizabeth Gould of Princeton University reported that each day's memories might be recorded in the neurons generated that day. Our brain might be going through daily renewal and change. White matter, the predominant matter in the brain, renews itself faster than grey matter. Grey matter just covers the surface of the cortex. While all these changes are going on in the brain, the rest of your body is also changing and renewing itself.

The youngest part of our body is our intestines that are 2-3 days old, while our taste buds replenish themselves every ten days. Then within weeks, our skin and lungs completely replenish themselves (2-4 weeks). Every few months our liver is replaced (5 months) and nails (6-10 months). Then every four months, after traveling more than 300 miles and going through the heart 170,000 times, 60 times per hour–our red blood cells are discarded, replaced by newly-created replacement cells. Our annual makeover includes new hair—for those that have hair (every 3-6 years), new bones (every 10 years), and lastly, most of our heart (every 20 years). The question arises why then, do we look so old if we are only 11 years of age?

As we renew each organ in our body—and we chronologically age—the rate of change decreases and we get more errors in the replacement cells. Many possible reasons could account for this—from the effects of natural radiation from the environment, to internal radiation from free radicals, to local physical damage and injuries—all could apply. It could be that our genetic material gathers faulty changes and its information becomes gradually degraded. Like a cassette tape that is repeatedly copied, or taking a photocopy of a photocopy where the image will eventually degrade.

It could also be that cells themselves become less efficient at cleaning up after themselves, leaving behind a lot of cellular trash. It could be that our stem cells—that exist even in older adults—eventually become less efficient with age as they are bombarded with toxins, harmful rays and temperature changes. Sometimes, when we damage an organ—for example damaging our lungs by smoking—the scarring tissue cannot be renewed and replaced. In effect, we stop our body from staying young.

This is why looking younger also means that you are also biologically younger and live longer. In the Danish Twin Study, Axel Skytthe and his colleagues reported that among monozygotic twins who share the same genes—the twin that looked younger is more likely to live longer. But there are no shortcuts. Undergoing plastic surgery does not result in longer life. There is also the Hayflick Limit with each of our 37.2 trillion cells in our body having a time bomb. At some point the cells reach their own individual lifespan and stop replicating.

The fact that we can measure aging using different metrics opens up a host of misunderstanding. We have seen that for individuals, chronological age is different from biological age. We also have a different method of measuring aging for populations. Demography—the study of patterns of populations—has a number of constructs to describe population aging, from lifespan to life-expectancy. Those promoting the search for immortality readily confuse constructs to give the impression that humans are living longer. Although as a population (demography) we are living longer we are not seeing this on an individual level (biology). How can this be?

How science tricks us into this confusion is the theme of this chapter. This concluding chapter will be discussing why increases in life-expectancy are not the same as living longer because one is based on populations and the other is based on individuals; that while the concept of immortality resides in our psychology the aim to living-longer resides in science and the two are unrelated; that the science of living longer involves a broader definition of our biology including our resident micro-organisms whereas in contract our attempts to extend life remain fixed on a cure-all approach. This conclusion highlights these inconsistencies, and offers a preview of what the future for immortality entails: a broader understanding of our evolution and our biology and how the symphony that we are dancing to is our own psychology.

Lifespan

Lifespan is described by The Oxford English dictionary as "the length of time for which a person or animal lives or a thing functions." Pragmatically, lifespan is defined as the longest period a member of a species has ever lived—this is Maximum Lifespan. Scientists have not yet determined what the maximum length of time that a human can live. This active theoretical field is home to lively speculation among gerontologists. When it comes to humans, the oldest person who has ever lived defines our lifespan. Verified by the Guinness World Records and the Gerontology Research Group, *Jeanne Louise Calment*, a French woman from Arles, France lived to 122 years and 164 days. Since her death in 1997, this age at death remains the definition of human lifespan. Lifespan is an outlier—an extreme case of longevity. It is different from other concepts such as longevity, mean life span, average life span, life expectancy, individual lifespan, average age of death, average life expectancy, modal age of death, modal age and median age of death.

In the anti-aging business, because our life-expectancy continues to improve, the New Age immortalists are arguing that we are living longer, that we are already pushing back the barriers of mortality. These declarations preach the mantra that it is only a matter of time before we start breaking all the hurdles that stop us from living forever—or at least to allow us to live for 130-150 years. A deception promoted by confusing individual aging with population aging.

Another problem exists with estimating age at very old age. In 1986, given continued reports of claims of extreme age, Norris and Ross McWhirter, the editors of *The Guinness Book of World Records*, noted the need to validate such assertions when they stated: "No single subject is more obscured by vanity, deceit, falsehood and deliberate fraud than the extremes of human longevity." Inaccuracy increases the older a person is reported to be. Stephen Coles reports how the U.S. Census Bureau dropped its estimate of centenarians from 2,700 in 1990 to 1,400 centenarians in 2000 after checking the dates of birth against claimed ages with the Social Security Administration. However, even this conservative number was inflated with 139 persons aged 110 or older. A truer number, based on physicians' estimates are more likely to be between 75 and 100 persons over the age of 110 years. If there is a problem with self-reporting age, subsequent problems arise with our interpretation.

Gerontologists have multiple ways of measuring individual aging: Chronological, functional, physiological and predictive (how many years you are expected to live.) These are very different, in contrast to population aging, which is defined by the percentage of older adults (60 or 65 plus) within a population. The tipping point comes when the older adult population reaches 10-13% of the total population. But this level is arbitrary and hides the fact that once a population starts aging—having fewer children rather than living longer—then the trend continues and unlikely to be reversed. Unless there are great social and economic upheavals, once a population starts to age then it gets increasing older.

It is a fallacy to assume that the "success story" of people living longer creates population aging, however intuitive that sounds. The primary reason for an aging population is a reduction in the number of children being born. This single factor determines an aging population, while living longer plays a very minor and statistically inconsequential role. In the U.S. in the last 100 years, the improvement in life expectancy at age 65 was only 5.7 years. This small improvement is not to be scoffed at, but it is not enough to cause the demographic revolution that we are witnessing today. If the number of births remained stable and mortality among children remained unchanged, the increase in an aging population because of this improvement in life-expectancy would be minimal. In reality, the sharp decline in births in all industrialized countries after the Second World War caused an imbalance. Because of good public health—clean water and safe food—most babies are surviving childhood. Early childhood vaccinations then allow most of these infants to reach adulthood and much later become older-adults. So that by 2050, in the U.S., the proportion of the 65 year and older population (15.6 percent) will be more than double that of children under age 5 (7.2 percent). This has serious repercussions. But for us the data helps to elucidate that an aging population is determined by the decline in births. Eventually, our overall populations will decline, despite the fears that we are over-populating. We are, as a population, exhibiting characteristics of extinction. A telling statistic does not come from demography but from the sale of diapers. In 2012, in Japan adult incontinence pants outsold baby nappies for the first time. By 2025, within most of our lifetimes, this same transformation will be occurring throughout most of the industrialized world.

Individual aging and population aging are two very different events and have very little effect on each other. The problem arises when biologists use population aging to support their argument, and vice versa, when demographers use biology to reinforce their prediction. Such errors become especially evident when the discussion turns to immortality, since these over-generalizations become magnified. However, because the areas of biology and demography are shrouded in technical terms, most of these mistakes are hidden from the public.

Life Expectancy

Look up "Life Expectancy" in dictionaries and they provide the wrong definition. It is not "the average number of years that a person or animal can expect to live" (Merriam Webster Dictionary, 2015). The only average we can get is average age at death—which might be what we are looking for, but does not translate well. Life expectancy is a median, a statistic, where half a cohort (born within a specific period of time) is expected to die before that age, and the other half will survive beyond that period. "Beyond that period" can mean to infinity. This statistic is not an average (mathematical mean) it is a mid-point. It is important to make this distinction because a median completely ignores extreme values—dying early in childhood or living to 110 years old. Unlike "average" (mathematical mean) that is sensitive to these extremes., life expectancy is not influenced by the maximum lifespan. Median, as a statistic, is impervious to outliers like lifespan. If all the people that live beyond their life expectancy—say 81 years of age—then continue live to 1,000 years old—the life expectancy statistics will not change. Such outliers do not affect the median. The median ignores scores that are very low and very high. This is the reason the median is used in gerontology—it gives us an indication of the average person and ignores those exceptional people that live up to and over 100 years of age—1 per 25,000—and those who die in infancy—6.15 per 1,000.

Gerontologists use life expectancy to define how populations age across history. The problem is that life expectancy is confused with lifespan. In 2002, Jim Oeppen and James Vaupel from the Max Planck Institute for Demographic Research showed that life expectancy in some of the world's developed countries (including Chile) has been increasing steadily by about 2.5 years per decade since the mid-19th century. They omit contradictory evidence from across the world, including a large country like Russia. Their argument that life expectancy is constantly improving also ignores latest life expectancy figures from industrialized countries that show an unexpected dip in life-expectancy. Despite this reality, there is no denying that long-term stable decline in mortality suggests a continued rise in life expectancy. However, in the long-term, this does not mean that such increases are linear or that the end point has moved—lifespan has remained static.

Even though there will be more centenarians both in terms of numbers—prevalence, because we have a larger population—and also in terms of percentage—incidence, because of improved public health—this does not mean that the lifespan has improved. Lot more people will reach adulthood but there is still a ceiling in terms of how old we can live to, that has not changed. Centenarians are exceptional beings and the reality is that most humans will not survive to age 100. Even for those that live to 100, the likelihood that they survive to become supercentenarians (110 years and older) is 1 in 6 million. As Fanny Janssen and his colleagues in the Netherlands reported, at some point, there will be a wall both biological and psychological. Very few people survive beyond 110. Worldwide, fewer than 50 people at any one time can claim such an honor.

Studies that show continuing increases in life expectancy cannot be used to argue that there is no lifespan, or that the lifespan can be increased. The statistic necessary to measure lifespan is age at death. That is just what Juliana da Silva Antero-Jacquemi from the Institute of Biomedical and Epidemiology Research in Sport, France, and her colleagues did. They analyzed 19,012 Olympian competitors and 1,205 supercentenarians—who live up to 110 years— that died between 1900 and 2013. Although most Olympians had longer life expectancy than the general population, they did not live as long as supercentenarians. However, they identified a common death trend between Olympians and centenarians—indicating similar mortality pressures over both populations that increase with age. The authors argue that a biological "barrier" model better explains mortality trend. They argue that there is a static lifespan. If life-expectancy is an inaccurate indicator of population aging then a better measure would be the age of death.

Modal Age of Death

Abraham de Moivre defined "expectation of life" in 1725 to mean just that, the likelihood that that a newborn has a 50-50 chance of living to a certain age. He arrived at this statistic in his work with survival curves. These are life tables that record the mortality of a given population. Life expectancy was not meant to be an all-encompassing statistic, applied to monitor aging populations, because as we have seen, it would be the wrong statistic. At the first International Congress of Demography held in Paris in 1878, the German statistician Wilhelm Lexis gave a paper in French entitled "On the normal length of human life and on the theory of the stability of statistical ratios." This followed the earlier theoretical works of the Belgian astronomer and mathematician Lambert Adolphe Jacques Quetelet in 1835. Clearly, great interest existed for defining an underlying unified theory of mortality. This statistic—the modal age of death—has come to be represented as M. This is the most common age of death—much better indication of how old a population is getting.

Both the life expectancy and the M have been increasing since the turn of the century. Interestingly, life expectancy was increasing faster than M because more children were surviving. If we imagine two lines from left to right, one line is at a steeper angle pointing up, while a second line has a slower incline. The two lines will eventually meet up on the right, meaning that most people survive to older ages and that most people are reaching a similar maximum year of death. But *M* has a much more complex story.

Väinö Kannisto has shown that across time, as the age of death increases slowly, the difference between the most common age of death and the outliers—those that live the longest—has become shorter. More people are reaching the maximum than the maximum moving higher. It seems that there is a wall around 110 years old and although many people are approaching this limit, the limit still exists. This is known as the compression of mortality, where death becomes bunched around a maximum. We do not see the maximum being pushed further out, meaning that the lifespan is relatively stable.

From this review there is one very definitive outcome that emerges. We are not living much longer and that there is a very hard barrier that stops us from living longer than 110 years. All other demographic evidence showing otherwise is relying on possibilities rather than probabilities. Any discussion of immortality has to rely on possibilities rather than probabilities. And possibilities remain outside of the realm of science.

Immortality and the science of living longer are two separate constructs. One is in the realm of science and probabilities, and the other is in the realm of religion and possibilities. We are at a tipping point in making this breakthrough in understanding this duality.

Homo Duplex

The French sociologist Emil Durkheim proposed that humans are "homo duplex," leading a double existence; one is rooted in biology and the other one in a social world. This interpretation afforded amazing foresight at the time. While our social self—morally, intellectually, and spiritually—is moving toward a more narcissistic form of individualism, in contrast our understanding of biology is moving in the opposite direction, showing how biologically diffuse we are.

Emil Durkheim argued that there would be a conflict between the biological and the social aspects of the homo duplex. We can argue that the conflict has started by addressing the belief in immortality: the narcissistic (belief in immortality) versus the collective (our biology).

On one side resides a narcissistic quest for the holy grail of immortality and on the other side the increasingly complex and collective biological world that we live in. The tipping point will come when we accept our destiny as a symphony of micro-organisms that responds to an ever changing environment. What Durkheim could not have predicted is that the search for immortality makes us more narcissistic while our biology makes us more collective.

Narcissism

The idea that we can become immortal requires that we believe we are special and deserve not to die, akin to god. For oligarchs such beliefs are the next step from their current sense of importance. But surprisingly most of us are also acquiring this sense of entitlement. Jean Twenge and Keith Campbell's exploration of the narcissistic epidemic document an alarming rise of narcissism at every level of our society. With the social media populated by a world of egos, our individualistic selves are flourishing. Among the oligarchs, there has always been godlike behavior. Traditionally oligarchs have already discovered immortality by transferring their wealth down through bequeathing their wealth to successive family members. Their individualism will live into eternity through the management of their wealth. These are not delusions of grandeur nowadays their search for immortality takes just another form. Such ambitions have always been with us. Historically we saw Gilgamesh's quest for the plant of immortality, the first emperor of China sending Xu Fu for the secret of immortality, and Francis Bacon experimenting with cryonics to expose the elixir of life—all of these were different methods in the search for immortality. The modern method might be science and technology but the quest continues unchanged. What has changed is the public's perceived access to this search. That anyone can benefit for progress—despite our awareness that health benefits (be they clean water or a heart transplant) are not accessible to all equally. This form of individualism has infected the general public, we are all behaving like gods.

Rousseau's 'Malo periculosam libertatem quam quietum servitium" says if gods were people, they would govern themselves democratically. In our mental model, the world is predictable and just, a true democracy. Despite an onslaught of daily news informing us otherwise, we still believe in a just world. We continue to be surprised by disasters or catastrophes, thinking that they are exceptions. They are not. They are exceptions only in our model of the world—the one that we cultivate in our head, the virtual box—because in our mind everything is in harmony, everything is balanced, and just. We continue to aspire to a world where we can "eliminate" death, "regain" youth, "fight" terrorism, "save" humanity and "cure" aging. These are illogical and delusional aims only if you are <u>not</u> a god. If we aspire to behave like, or think that we are gods, then these aspirations are attainable. These aspirations confer a delusional sense of control over our world. How did we get here?

Our Selfish Sense of Self

In our mind, in our model of how the world operates, we have a causal model of the world that requires that immortality remains a central feature as it allows us not to confront death. The model we have built in our mind is reliant on constancy, order and logic. The sole purpose of having such a complex brain is to represent the world. Every day, we adjust this model so that we can better predict outcomes. Mostly this activity remains below conscious awareness and we only become aware when our brain requires our full attention in order to address some complex event.

Everyone's brain generates a model of the world, a virtual reality box that requires that you are the center of this universe. All animals do this to varying degrees of complexity. There is even a representation of you that exists physically along the cortex that runs from ear to ear. This the thin layer of grey matter covering the brain, has a representation of the body, a *homunculus* Latin for "Little Man."

The *homunculus* includes both a sensory as well as a motor representation of the divisions of the body. It is extremely sensitive to learning, so that if you are learning to read braille the *homunculus* will grow that cortical part where the fingers are represented. The rest of the brain similarly changes. Some parts change every day, while others are more resistant to change. Our interaction in our environment determines where the growth will take place but we are still at the center of this mental universe. It is easy to see how we start to think like gods. This unconscious model of the world furnishes us with a feeling of mastery and control because we can predict and effect change. It is the conscious part of our brain that remains problematic to understand.

It began when scientists started finding that conscious thought is a product of an unconscious process. We are "aware" because of an earlier process that we are not aware of that wants us to be aware. The late Benjamin Libet from University of California in San Francisco was a pioneer in showing that a conscious decision can be monitored neurologically—sometimes as much as ten seconds before the activity appears—which he termed readiness potential. In effect, by monitoring the brain's electrical activity we can predict rudimentary activity before people become conscious of it, such as moving your index finger. More recently, Itzak Fried from University of California in Los Angeles recorded single neurons and found that the readiness potential isn't a diffuse state of readiness, but a very specific set of instructions. Our consciousness was an afterthought to a specific decision that has already been taken. This resulted in what Daniel Wegner called in his 2002 book, *The Illusion of Conscious Will.* The fundamental principle of our thinking is that we have control. We are at the center of our model and are not actors on a stage but directors of our legacy. We need conscious will because our large brain demands this selfish control, while other animals do not need this illusion.

Some animals, like humans, have a very complex, symbolic and scientific/mathematical models while other animals have a more simplified survival-level model. Our unique ability to project a future requires us to develop a sense of progress through time—but not far enough to acknowledge our death. In most cases this creates a problem since we do not have anything planned for "after retirement." The future that we design for ourselves become our narrative arc—a unified mental narrative about our story.

Because in our narrative arc we learn to look outward for validation, our narcissism becomes misplaced and our collective reality takes over.

Narrative Arc

Our big brain provides us with lifespan expectations, an evolving story line. By continually re-interpreting that past in order to validate the present and to propel us towards our anticipated future. We expect to grow up healthy, get a job, maybe marry or have kids, buy or have a house, be established, successful, and then retire and slow down. Each individual has different trajectories and nuances, but the general flow of our narrative remains the same and it makes for some interesting anomalies. We accept our fate easily when reality matches our internal narrative arc.

A 58-year-old woman was misdiagnosed with Alzheimer's disease. Despite having no real expression of the disease and with the diagnosis made purely random by a disturbed neurologist, the patient was deeply convinced that the diagnosis was correct, even when she was confronted with contradictory evidence. But this was part of her narrative arc. Her mother had dementia and she expected to get dementia. She trusted the neurologist and therefore the diagnosis corroborated her narrative arc. In this sense, the diagnosis was not a neutral piece of information. It reinforced an expectation. She might have had other issues, maybe emotional ones, but the need to tell a story, to have a coherent narrative overwhelms the reality of the situation. The consequences of a diagnosis—whether valid or not— may be similar to persistent false memories or stereotypes. And we internalize some stereotypes so much that we acquiesce to expectations.

Our narrative arc also determines when we die. Within our narrative, significant days are psychological anchors. They can either act as a lifeline or a deadline. David Phillips, with the University of California San Diego, has been looking at this phenomenon for some time. In 1992 Phillips and his colleagues examined deaths from natural causes in two samples of around three million people. Women are more likely to die in the week following their birthdays than in any other week of the year. The frequency of female deaths dips below normal just before their birthday. It seems that females are able to prolong life briefly until they have reached a positive, symbolically meaningful occasion. For women a birthday seems to function as a "lifeline." In contrast, male deaths peak shortly before their birthday, suggesting that the birthday functions as a "deadline" for males. In their narrative arc, at older ages men are more likely to portray their looming birthday as a negative sign. The importance of a "lifeline" or a "deadline" also works for other significant days.

David Phillips and Elliot King showed that in a small Jewish group death declines by about a third below normal before the Jewish holiday of Passover and then peaks by the same amount the week after. It seems that Jewish people hold on to life a little bit longer to celebrate Passover. Since the date of Passover changes each year, this effect is not seasonal or related to other external variables, but more likely be caused by how the narrative arc includes sharing Passover with family. In contrast, non-Jewish mortality showed no such pattern around the same period.

Others have different psychological anchors that determine when they are more likely to die. David Phillips again, this time with Daniel Smith looked at when Chinese die. They found that Chinese people die less by a third the week before the Harvest Moon Festival and peaks by the same amount the week after. Same as for Jews and Passover, Chinese hold on to life to experience the Moon Festival. This is known as the Hound of the Baskervilles effect, where psychological stress determines the timing of death.

Such timing of death is perplexing. Does the narrative arc truly influence when we die or is there a simpler answer? There could be behaviors around this period that either relax or stress the individual. Such stresses might explain why deaths in the West spike during Christmas and New Year's holiday period. This increased deaths persists after adjusting for trends and seasons and seems to be growing proportionately larger over time. More people are dying around these periods of festivities in industrialized countries. Not only are these periods stressful and indulgent, there is also the possibility that people delay seeking medical treatment while entertaining or being entertained. Medical and emergency services might also not be as efficient during holiday periods. There are also excesses of behavior and diet during these periods. So, we cannot definitively say that these days are important enough for us to "will" to die or not. But under certain situations, the will to die becomes a strong contender.

Tetraphobia, the practice of avoiding instances of the number "4" is a superstition that is common in China, Taiwan, Singapore, Malaysia, Japan, Korea and Vietnam. This superstition seems to have arisen from the similarity of the pronunciation of the word "four" and "death" in Mandarin, Cantonese, and Japanese. This phobia surpasses our own Western superstition of triskaidekaphobia relating to the number 13. Similarly, tetraphobia results in the number four being omitted in floor and room assignment in hospitals and hotels, in numbering of new houses and in such mundane identification as car park spaces. This practice seems to have followed Asian immigrants to Canada to the chagrin and pushback of firefighters. David Phillips again has provided evidence for this when by looking at death from heart disease among Chinese and Japanese Americans. What he found was that there are one in twelve extra deaths among Chinese and Japanese Americans on the fourth of the month. No such increases showed up among other populations. Death increases on psychologically significant days. If our narrative arc includes an expectation that we will die on a certain day, we are likely to honor that expectation.

What if the narrative arc of our death is interfered with? We know that at some predetermined age, most likely to mirror our parents' death, we will die. As the date becomes a reality there are certain days such as our birthdate that we look forward to as an accomplishment (for women) or as a deadline (for men.) Some festivities which are stressful, are likely to hasten our demise (Christmas and New Year) while other holidays we hold back till after they ass (Passover for Jews and Harvest Moon Festival for Chinese.) Then there are days that we have a phobia of dying that acts as a self-fulfilling prophecy. Our narrative arc is more than a script that we follow. It is writing the story of life as we live it and we have some control over when to give up or try that little harder.

We fall in step with our internal narrative. We hold dual ideas about getting older. We know intellectually that we will die, but we conduct our day-to-day activities ignorant of this ultimate fate. The background belief of some avenue for immortality might be enough to deflect some of the fear of dying. But in contrast we hold a narrative arc, a storyline about how our lives will progress, and the best way our big brain develops this narrative arc is from other people.

Becca Levy with Yale University and her colleagues in 2000 primed—bring to awareness—both older and young participants with either negative or positive stereotypes of old age. Then they were asked them to respond to hypothetical medical situations involving fatal illnesses. They found that older participants who were primed with negative stereotypes were more likely to refuse life-prolonged interventions. Those primed with positive images tended to accept medical interventions. Younger participants showed no difference, indicating that the stereotypes had less relevance to them and did not influence them. Ageism can diminish older adults' will to live. Being reminded of the incapacity of older age hastened the need to end life. We are not born with our narrative arc. We learn what our story is from other people. We inherit a set of expectations especially when we are older and the expectations are negative. Simone de Beauvoir and later Robert Butler both talked about this ageism and how society tends to have a negative view of older people. This collective influence is internalized, especially if we believe that it applies to us. As with mirror neurons that we discussed in chapter 4, other people influence us more than we give them credit for. We can conclude that although our model of "self" is narcissist in contrast we function and live collectively.

Collective Self

Historically four philosophical thoughts shifted us away from being the center of the universe. Incrementally moving us away from perceiving the world and us as being at the center of the universe towards a more collective universe where we occupy a more peripheral position. The first such radical thinker shifted us away from mythology, and the notion that everything happens because " god wants it to happen." He was Thales of Miletus a 6th century BC philosopher who suggested that we should observe physical events without assigning the cause to "god." Such subtle change in focus gave birth to science and he is credited with being the father of science. As a result, we began to understand that a causal pattern exists in the world–that there are logical sequences that do not require the intervention of a central being. The development of science took us into amazing logical worlds that were previously hidden. We stopped ascribing everything to one entity and tried to observe other underlying laws of nature. Not one law (god), but multiple laws. However we still saw nature as revolving around us. This assurance of egocentric solidity was shattered in the early 1900s on three counts. Darwin reversed more than 5,000 years of thinking that we are separate and unique beings by showing how all animals are related—including humans. Darwin moved our perception of ourselves from a place of superiority to a place on a continuum. Around the same time, Sigmund Freud developed the concept of an unconscious mind. He exposed that a part of us hid events and feelings from our consciousness—such as the Oedipus complex, libido and death drive, among others. Freud's main contribution was the acceptance that our conscious self is but a component of who we are. We do not know all of "us," we have a reality hidden from us. What Freud did for psychology, Albert Einstein then did for our concept of reality and the universe. Einstein, a theoretical physicist, developed a general theory of relativity that together with quantum mechanics and the law of the photoelectric effect evolved into quantum theory. Einstein transformed Newtonian mechanics—where objects were treated as physical representation but much smaller— to one where at great microscopic details, these realities changed into energy and shivering mass of probabilities. He conceived of the world as composed of waves of energy, a vibrating nexus of excited mass that even change time welcome to the universe of relativity.

These ideas came from a culmination of *a priori* small developments that helped Thales, Darwin, Freud and Einstein make these conceptual leaps. Moving towards a collective universe and leaving behind a narcissistic view of the world explains our conundrum with immortality.

As part of our survival strategy—our K-strategy where we invest heavily in a few children—developing a large brain comes with longevity. A big brain and longevity go together since longevity enables us time to impart this accumulated knowledge to the next generation. But there was a down side to this strategy. Our big brain had to accept the awareness of our eventual death. But this throws the model of our world into disarray. To diminish this fear, we developed multiple tricks of the mind. These tricks are reliant on a fundamental premise that there is constancy in the world. The lynchpin of this constancy—expressed as a fair world, orderly and logical—is that everything will remain constant. In our mind it is difficult for us to conceive that we will die, age, become incapacitated, become blind, deaf or incarcerated. And the belief in immortality, expressed through tricks of our psychology—such as having a soul, a legacy, cryonics, over optimism of health benefits and engineering health—is at the center of this belief. We deny that we will eventually be no more since our model of the world cannot explain it. For this model to function it has to assume that we are at the center of our universe, a narcissistic imperative. But this is not true. Thales, Darwin, Freud and Einstein have shown us how our perception of the universe and ourselves is incomplete and pushing us away from use being the center of the universe. The next frontier is to question the idea of self to explore a more collective form of "self."

Both our psychology and our biology are intertwined with a social world and with the environment. We negotiate our reality with people and the environment around us. On one side is the concept of "me"—the narcissistic self—and on the other the story of "others"—our collective existence. The reality is that there is a place where there such a distinction does not exist. Our body holds that special place. It is both part of the environment and part "me." This argument gains importance because, as we have already seen, our biology and our psychology cannot be separated from the environment.

My environment, community, family and friends can determine my behavior and outcomes, as much as I think I do myself. My interaction with the world leaves evidence in my genes, just as I leave traces in my geography and environment. Such a symbiotic relationship exposes humans to a greater sense of belonging within their geography since we carry our community in our bodies. In Lawrence Durrell's novel *Justine*, the narrator says that "we are the children of our landscape; it dictates behavior and even thought in the measure to which we are responsive to it."

If we are going to understand how extreme-longevity develops, we need to understand this construct much better than we do today. On the whole, we have discarded the idea that we age because we invested our resources in our genes and left no resources for maintaining our body or mind. That nature did not engineer aging but that aging is what happens when the engineering runs out has become a simplistic and erroneous interpretation of the sophistication of nature. In contrast biologists have come to see aging as an adaptive feature, a strategy for survival. We need to learn more about what adaptive features aging brings. In the most obvious way, aging allows for an investment in educating and nurturing the young. But there is more as we have learned in our exploration of immortality. Our biology changes to adapt to our environment. Plasmids continue to interact with our genome as we age. Genetic changes continue into older ages and aging is part of the engineering. Because aging has survived, then it seems that aging has meaning. We just do not fully understand this meaning. By looking at aging the way nature does we might be able to understand this meaning.

The science of aging still needs to develop more than just promoting health to assure longer life. Eating good quality food, moderate consumption of (red) wine, and enjoying the company of friends is not only good for longevity, but define some of life's pleasures. We do not need science to tell us that. We have a short lease on life. If we use it wisely and cultivate quality, it will eventually contribute to the quantity of life as well. But there is more to aging and the search for immortality has shown us some avenues that we need to explore. "Homo duplex" highlights a conflict between who we think we are and who we truly are. We have on one side the belief in constancy and order with immortality acting as an anchor that keeps this worldview in order. And on the other hand the appreciation of our biological diversity and interconnectedness with an every changing environment. Change versus constancy, this is the "homo-duplex" that we are experiencing today.

Immortality vs. Longer Life

Appreciating that longevity is intimately connected with our environment, with other "homo-sapiens micro-organisms" then our view of longevity changes. Staying healthy relates to how well we maintain a balance with our environment—developing immunology, safe environment, built resilience, supportive diet and activity. A balance maintained both through our history of development—how appropriately we were prepared in the womb for the outside world, and our subsequent "match" with our environment— and our biological capacity— genes, epi-genes, and our micro-organism symbionts and environmental conditions, the "Makeham" constant.

Such conditions establish a trajectory, a certain capacity for flexibility and a degree of plasticity. Plasticity refers to the body's short-term capacity for improvement or decline. It is no longer a matter of tweaking a gene here and there, but appreciating our trajectory in life. Both where we start in life and changes that are made along the way contribute to our health and longevity. In most cases, behaviors and events make small adjustments—negative and positive—to this trajectory. Sometimes they promote health and longevity, and sometimes they cause trauma and disease. Such changes are important in how our bodies adapt to the environment. However, it seems that such an intimate relationship with the environment become compromised as we get older. Looking at the environment might hold clues as to why that is.

Restricted Travel

The constant exposure to different environmental micro-organisms—in the food we eat, water we drink and air we breathe, creates an environmental assault. Through hormesis our body—including our plasmids and micro-organisms—build antibodies. Extremely long-lived individuals usually stay in one place, the place where they were born. The island Blue Zones are not easily accessible places, and few of the centenarians travelled away from their village. The positive outcomes for restricted travel provide us with a clue.

In industrialized countries, we tend to travel more, become infected with more microbes to which our bodies must adapt, constantly changing our immune system. Not being immune to travel-related diseases, we tend to suffer more from stomach bugs, fever, and breathing problems—especially after travelling to Central America, South Central Asia, Northeast Asia, and North Africa. In 1998 (the most recent data), there was a daily movement of 1.4 million persons occurred worldwide, which the U.S. Institute of Medicine blamed as the principal factor contributing to the global emergence of infectious diseases. After a visit to developing countries, one in seven travelers report some health problems–especially those visiting friends and family. This scenario does not include the much larger influence of other travelers visiting us from developing countries, leading to greater exposure and infection. Unless there is an influenza epidemic, which brings travel to a stop, we are unlikely to take much notice. How infections affect older people, especially after travel or coming in contact with people who have travelled remains a mystery.

The fact that centenarians tend to live with other centenarians, as in the Blue Zones, suggests that there might be an additional social component. Similar to the Roseto effect excessive stress in life becomes counterbalanced by a sense of tribe and community. A feeling that someone has your back has significant health benefit. Being economically secure might also provide such support, and again, like the Roseto effect, this remains subjective. Be content with your lot whatever your lot is.

This again reinforces how multiple factors influence longevity. But despite the success of centenarians and supercentenarians, their death reinforces the existence of an absolute limit on life. Lifespan is real. The question is how this is brought about. The dramatic change in gut bacteria from adults to centenarians and then supercentenarians provides a clue as to what might be happening. The evolution of bacteria might have positive effects in younger ages but deleterious effects as we age. We have seen this type of dual role with genes, where the beneficial effect is expressed early while the negative effect comes much later. This concept of antagonistic pleiotropy might also apply to bacteria. When in 2014 Martin Blaser and Glenn Webb proposed that bacteria kill older adults, they might not have far off from what we are observing. The question then would it be possible then to change the bacteria to promote longevity? And again we fall into the fountain of youth narrative, of trying to find a panacea to aging. Although we seem to have other checks on our mortality—such as our telomeres and stem cell depletion—by all accounts our lifespan can be much longer. Just changing the bacteria might increase our potential for longer life but scientific evidence points us away from simple solutions however. Our evolving knowledge of aging paints a more nuanced and interdependent picture. Changing one aspect of this balance will not bring about comprehensive change. The first order of business should be to understand the psychology of immortality in order to move beyond the search for binary answers.

Collective Beings

The more we look at our body, the more we appreciate that we are made up of collective organisms. Simone de Beauvoir, in her 1949 book *The Second Sex,* said it best when she observed that "The body is not a thing, it is a situation: it is our grasp on the world and our sketch of our project." Our bodies and our brain are not exclusive entities—we have parts of other organisms and other people within us. In addition to our genes that we inherit from various sources, there are viruses, bacteria and potentially, other human cells within our body. Even our genes and brain are not deterministic and are influenced by external events.

Our body is home to a universe of external components. Not only is it permeable to outside organisms, our brain is similarly influenced by external events–both in terms of how it functions and how it behaves. We have specialized areas in our brain that "mirror" our environment. Genes also exist, genes that are operated by the environment through epigenetic influence and plasmids—jumping genes. Richard Rorty in 1979 said this beautifully " . . . had physiology been more obvious, psychology would never have arisen—can be reaffirmed. Indeed, we can strengthen it and say that if the body had been easier to understand, nobody would have thought that we had a mind." (p. 239).

Conclusion

Immortality means controlling our environment from before birth to forever. Even if we eliminate the "forever" from this equation, and restrict it to a normal lifetime, controlling the environment would be a monumental and uncharted task. We will have to control and determine the as-yet-unknown effects of trillions of micro-organisms that inhabit us and our immediate environment, how seasonal influences determine their growth, our resilience to them, how genes are exchanged with twins, siblings, and with our children, how environmental conditions determine the function of these genes. We have to learn why and how plasmids change positions on our chromosomes, why they infect us and who controls this behavior. We need to control those areas of our brain designed to mimic other people's behavior or control other people's behavior. We have to control other people that we interact with, restrict our exposure to novel micro-organisms (or maybe just specific ones)—all of which we are just now starting to understand. Even if we had the necessary knowledge, it becomes a surreal task to control this environment for immortality.

And when we have finished all of this, then we have to make sure that no unforeseen trauma, iatrogenic calamities–a wrong step or an errant accident befalls us. Our genes might already be immortal, but our bodies are disposable and vulnerable. From this discussion the construct of immortality emerges very clearly as a purely psychological construct. This realization, that we are addressing a psychological desire, provides us with a better focus. We want to remain as we are today. Or better still, we do not want change. This is a very different psychological concept from desiring immortality. Immortality is a side effect of not wanting to change.

But change is how our longevity is preserved. Since our adaptation to the environment changes our genes our immunology. Interacting with our environment, although detrimental to the body, is beneficial for our genes and for our survival as a species. Aging is a positive method of changing our genetic expression by interacting with and adapting to our environment. In the process of this interaction, we become less resilient and eventually cells— having successfully modified our genes for future generations—start to die off. This, then, might be the symphony that Sherwin Nuland in *How We Die* talks about. Because dying cells secrete chemicals that disrupt other cells in their immediate environment, even a small percentage of dying cells can have a much broader domino effect on neighboring cells. There is a tipping point before "…we implode into eternity." This logic goes against the business of aging and makes the search for immortality a search for the Holy Grail, more fiction than science, more religion than fact. We cannot have immortality since it goes against our strategy for survival as a species. Our mortality teaches us that we are a part of a bigger meaning. We are connected with those around us and with the universe we inhabit. Our short lease on life is our window to gaze upon this wonder.

∞

INDEX

Information from the author:

I am a tenured professor of gerontology and I receive no funding from federal or state governments and have no invested interest in aging research. I welcome any comments and criticisms. You can contact me at the following:

drmariusgarrett@gmail.com

Or you can write to me at:

PO Box 331
La Mesa, CA 91944
USA

You can view my full biographical profile at:

https://sites.google.com/site/mariodrmariogarrettcom/

Mario D. Garrett